I WISH SOMEONE HAD TOLD ME...

I WISH SOMEONE HAD TOLD ME...

195 THINGS YOU MUST KNOW BEFORE YOU HAVE YOUR BABY (BUT EVEN YOUR BEST FRIEND WON'T DARE TO TELL YOU)

UNSPOKEN TRUTHS ABOUT WHAT REALLY HAPPENS TO WOMEN DURING LABOUR, CHILDBIRTH AND THE FIRST FEW WEEKS OF MOTHERHOOD

DR JENNIFER HACKER PEARSON PhD

POWERED by FEAR
PUBLISHING

AUTHOR NOTE:

While every care has been taken in researching and compiling the medical information in this book, it is in no way intended to replace or supersede professional medical advice. Neither the author nor the publisher may be held responsible for any action or claim howsoever resulting from the use of this book or any information contained in it. Readers must obtain their own professional medical advice before relying on or otherwise making use of the medical information contained in this book.

Powered by Fear Publishing, Sydney, Australia
www.DrJen.com.au

Text copyright © Jennifer Hacker Pearson 2016. Updated 2022
Designed by Luke Causby at Blue Cork
Typeset in Bembo
ISBN 978-0-9954212-0-2 (paperback)
ISBN 978-0-9954212-1-9 (E-book)

I would just like to mention that I am eternally grateful to the group of midwives at the Royal Hospital for Women who helped bring all three of my babies into the world. Midwives and obstetricians do an amazing job. I am in no way criticising them or any of the various birth guides/manuals/books/videos/DVDs and whatever else is on the market. *I Wish Someone Had Told Me...* is compiled of true experiences which mothers wish they had been told about before they had their baby. This book is not encouraging women in any direction pre- or post-birth. The following accounts are merely personal experiences.

ACKNOWLEDGEMENTS

This book would not exist without the contribution, encouragement, openness and support from the hundreds of mums that told me their stories. Most I had never met before but by the end we were all connected through motherhood. I appreciate the time you took to share your stories with me and the level of detail you went in to. I hope you like the finished product.

There are many people that have supported me since the book's infancy. Thank you! Without you I am not sure I ever would have got it off the ground. I would especially like to mention the ladies from my three mothers' groups – thrown together by chance, you have become such wonderful friends and I am eternally grateful for your support, not only for the book but through my ups and downs of motherhood.

Thank you to Felicity Copeland, midwife extraordinaire, for your support and expertise. I wish every woman had the chance to have you as their midwife.

I would like to thank Dr Diane Rees, Kelly Wilmott, Jess Beaton, Erik Hamre and Sadie Jobling for their support and expertise in all things editing, proof-reading, publishing and designing.

A special thank you goes to Alfie Arcidiacono for his energy, support and introducing me to the right people to help turn the manuscript into an actual book.

I am indebted to Kate and Rod Power. Thank you for everything you have done for me. You took me under your big, experienced wing and taught me so much, never asking for anything in return. I am so grateful for your time, energy and support. I feel truly blessed to have met you.

Thank you to my friends and family, especially my three perfectly imperfect children – you are remarkable human beings who amaze and inspire me daily. I adore you and I thank you for enriching my life.

There are not enough thanks in the world for my literally longsuffering husband, without whom this book definitely would not have been written. Mainly, because he is part of the reason I have three kids, but also because he has been endlessly supportive, encouraging and involved. He has given me time and space to write (which is no mean feat with three little kids) and a kick up the butt when I needed it. Thank you. PS You're not really a knob.

For Everly, Daniel and Jake

PREFACE

Birth is not only about making babies. Birth is about making mothers – strong, competent, capable mothers who trust themselves and know their inner strength.

Barbara Katz Rothman

A long with a baby a mother is born. Becoming a mother is a transformation for every woman. It is known as *matrescence*. Yet, we don't talk about this life-changing developmental transformation. We don't tell women that they will change physically, psychologically, emotionally and spiritually. Imagine if you knew what other mothers already know about this life-changing time. Imagine how prepared you would feel. You would know that what you are experiencing is probably totally normal, and you would feel understood, heard and not alone.

I researched and wrote this book to prepare and empower mums to-be and new mothers. It is intended to give women information they probably won't find elsewhere but absolutely must know going into childbirth, matrescence and motherhood.

I struggled unbelievably when my third baby was born. I had three kids within three-and-a-half years, and my daughter's birth (well, her existence really) saw me battle like I had never before. Don't get me wrong, I love her dearly – I always have and always will – but I was on a rocky road, and suffering. I had already started writing *I Wish Someone Had Told Me…* after my first birth, with the intention of bringing the unspoken aspects of childbirth, and early motherhood to the surface in a light-hearted, entertaining way. However, when I managed to get some sanity back after my third birth (18 months after she was born!), I decided that I *must* publish this book ASAP. I was thinking about all the mums out there that were struggling like me – scared about childbirth, not understanding matrescence or what they are feeling, second-guessing their mothering, worrying and not thriving. Just surviving. I knew I had to publish this book to let women know what has happened to other mothers, and that they are not alone in their experiences.

If by empowering women with this knowledge I can help just one mum get through her challenging time, then my book as done its job.

I really want to stress that *I Wish Someone Had Told Me…* was not written to scare anyone. Too often truths about childbirth, matrescence and motherhood are skimmed over, dumbed down or conveniently forgotten to share. Not here! This book is the truth; warts and all. All the embarrassing, gross and funny things that can happen to women during labour, childbirth and the first few weeks of motherhood, told one humorous paragraph at a time. Over one thousand mothers have contributed their experiences, because like me, they want to tell it like it is and empower mums in the process.

I hold a PhD in Medicine, so you will find some medical facts throughout the book but primarily I wrote this book as a mother, for mothers. I have been there. I know how much you wonder if you are the only woman on earth to have *that* experience, or *those* feelings. I know you doubt and second-guess yourself (I still do, many years later!). That's why I wrote this book.

Knowledge is power. Empower yourself with information you probably won't hear elsewhere and be assured that these things do happen, they are normal, they are nothing to be scared of, there is nothing wrong with you, and there is a lighter side to it all. But mostly, you are not alone!

NB: I believe that as long as a child has a loving home environment, the setup of it is irrelevant. In this book, I use the term husband and insinuate a partner is male only because that is true for me.

INTRODUCTION

Maybe I was naive, but I thought that a straight-forward birth was the norm. You know, the ones they show you at antenatal class. Breathe, breathe, push, push and... "Congratulations, here is your baby!" Well, that was until my first *little* bundle-of-joy spectacularly, and traumatically, entered the world at 9lb 2oz (that's 4.2kg to all us youngens) and 22.5 inches (57cm!!!). I won't even mention the size of his head! It was the Big Kahuna of births, or at least so I thought. It all started December 22 at 4pm. My waters broke while I was placing a meticulously wrapped present under the Christmas tree (a lot of stuff was still meticulous back then. Nowadays I can't remember how to spell the word). After weeks of trying everything, and I mean *everything*, to get this baby out before Christmas (his due date was 16 December), I resigned to the fact that I would still be pregnant on Christmas Day. Just on a side note, I don't believe any of the "natural methods" to induce labour really work. Short of guzzling a castor oil concoction I had heard about, I did try it all (if you want any tips drop me a line). I drew the line at the castor oil; I was already miserable enough, and the thought of vomit and diarrhoea, without labour, was too much for me to bear. After three "late" babies, I am now a firm believer that your baby will come when it is good and ready.

So anyway, here I was squatting to place the present under the tree when I heard a *POP!* It really did sound like when you put your index finger inside your cheek and push it out. From my many hours research of Hollywood movies, I of course did not realise it was my waters. Weren't they meant to gush out? While you're in a supermarket or somewhere similarly embarrassing? "Clean up in aisle three, clean up in aisle three!"

Anyway, they did not gush (more about that later), in fact I could have mistaken it for normal girly fluid had I not been so desperately on the lookout for a sign that labour was imminent. I called my midwife and said "I think my waters have broken". She told me to put in a maternity pad and call her when it was full. Sure enough I was back on the phone to her 10 minutes later. She asked me to come in to check that the baby was OK and there was no meconium (baby poo) in the fluid. I was strangely calm now. For all the scenarios I had imagined in the 41 weeks leading up to this point, I even surprised myself with my level of serenity.

OK, better get to hospital... Oh, better call Hubs first. Still calm as anything I called my beloved and asked him if he wasn't too busy, would he mind coming home as my waters had broken and I needed to go to the hospital to check everything was alright (true story, these were my exact words). So I created myself a lovely garbage bag-covered cushion on the couch, plonked myself on that moist throne and waited for Hubs to arrive. Then it dawned on me. Something was missing. Wasn't I meant to have contractions!? Where were they? Am I having them and I wasn't realising? Broken waters equals onset of labour, right? Where on earth were my contractions? Yes, it did occur to me for a nanosecond that I may be the world's first woman who is going to give birth without any pain, but alas no (although I have since learnt I wouldn't be the first after all).

Contractions weren't missing. I was not in labour and I was sadly not Super-Mum to be. Waters can break without contractions!

We went to the hospital and got the all clear. Baby's fine, waters are clear, induction booked for 6am if labour doesn't start naturally overnight. Well, as exciting as that was, it also meant that Hubs and I didn't sleep a wink (actually I think he slept one wink but I rudely interrupted that). Apart from the concerto I was creating with my bum-on-garbage-bag band every time I rolled over (the waters just keep coming!) we couldn't sleep because we were excited, nervous, anxious etc. etc. etc.

Finally, at 3am I thought I felt something. I went to the bathroom and back to bed, back to the bathroom and back to bed. Into the bathroom and back to bed again. Well, you get the picture. I wasn't sure whether I should wake Hubs to tell him what I thought might be happening. I really should have scrapped that worry because my constant back and forth to the bathroom, never mind the piping up of the garbage-bag band every time I lay back in bed, woke him anyway. I told him that I thought maybe something was going on, so we got up and had a cup of tea (as you do!?!). It really didn't take long from there. By 6am I was in sufficient agony and called my midwife to let her know I'd be coming in soon. She told me to come in when I couldn't breathe through the contractions. Time went on, yadda yadda yadda, pain got worse, yadda yadda yadda, contractions three minutes apart, yadda yadda yadda, into car and off to hospital. This is where my worst fear came true (or at least I thought it was my greatest fear. My fears have somewhat changed since becoming a mum). Please keep in mind that I hadn't given birth at this point and all (well, the majority) of my pride and dignity were still intact. So really it was a silly thought to have, but… after so many antenatal appointments in the hospital and having walked in and out so many times, I thought: please dear Universe do not let me have a contraction in the foyer of the hospital. And of course I did. In the middle of the foyer, in what seemed like peak-hour, there I was groaning and moaning. Oh the embarrassment! Little did I know that I would look back on that moment as the catalyst of the day that stole my embarrassment for eternity (most things that would have embarrassed me pre-babies now leave me cold).

I did make it to the birth centre however, and upon examination was pleasantly surprised to be 8cm dilated. Woohoo, we're going to have our baby soon! Even my midwife said that she thinks the baby would be born soon and that Hubs didn't even have time to go back to the car to get my bag with the nice relaxation music, essential oils, blow-up pillow, string bikini and other mostly useless labouring paraphernalia I had amassed. So I laboured. I laboured hard. In the bath, on the bean bag, on the bed, on Hubs. The last 2cm really are the hardest. But I got there, and a short time after arrival I was pushing my little heart out. I pushed and I pushed and I pushed. The problem was I really didn't feel like pushing (warning bells!), but I did push. For two hours! Nothing was happening. Things were getting out of hand. The baby was getting distressed, my midwife was getting distressed, Hubs was getting distressed; I think I was the only person not getting distressed, or maybe I was and I was just too out of it to realise. My beta-endorphins (which kick-start our naturally occurring pain killers, aka our best friend) were in overdrive. Couple that with a sleepless night and Whoa Mumma, where was I again? My midwife had obviously notified the doctors because things changed rapidly (in hindsight I remember in antenatal class we were told that if your midwife presses *the red button* in your birthing suite there is trouble).

INTRODUCTION

As instructed, I waddled to the delivery suite. The 20 meters took me about 20 minutes as my contractions tumbled one on top of the other. They seemed continuous. I was begging Hubs and my midwife for an epidural. She kept assuring me that when the doctors came they would deliver the baby and I wouldn't need an epidural. Oh my, that was a tough hour. I was pacing, screaming, whimpering, begging, drifting in and out of consciousness. Finally, the doctors arrived. They placed my feet in stirrups and gave me a small local anaesthetic in my perineum (yes, that small space between hole one and hole two). This was the only pain medication I had throughout this whole adventure. I wished they could have given me a massive dose to numb my whole body and let me go to sleep (at that stage I would have even taken a mallet to the head). The next noise I heard was the metallic clinking of scissors as those two holes became one (well, almost). I was still having very strong and frequent contractions and I'd had the episiotomy, so where was my baby?

He was stuck. They tried the ventouse (suction cup) but even with all the obstetrician's might, and I'm talking leveraging a leg on the end of the bed and yanking with every muscle in her body (like in a bad comedy), the cup slipped off his head; three times! With forceps they finally managed to safely deliver his head but then his shoulders were stuck. As I said in the beginning, big baby! It was only a few weeks later, once he was safely in our home and the delivery was a not-nearly-distant-enough memory, that I found out he had a shoulder dystocia. Apparently it is an obstetrical emergency and often leads to foetal death because the head is out but the rest of the body is stuck. Yikes!

Anyway back to the story, out come the forceps. Holey moley

have you seen those things?

It hurt more than anything else I have ever experienced in my life. It felt like they were pulling my legs out of my hip sockets. I particularly remember my right hip. With every yank I thought my eyes would pop out of my head. It was excruciating, there are no words to describe how bad it was. But I made it. We both did. And hearing my son's first few cries was the sweetest sound in the world. To this day I believe I was a split second away from a caesarean. I also believe that not having had an epidural gave me the ability to assist by pushing while they were pulling. But I will never know and I don't really care, because like so many women before me it didn't mean a thing anymore now I was holding my child. The most precious thing on this earth; so fragile, small and gooey.

Awww, happy ending, right?

Unfortunately, not. After cuddling and feeding my boy for what seemed like five minutes, I was rushed away to theatre where I promptly received a spinal block to numb me from the waist down (thanks very much, I could have used that a few hours earlier!) and was stitched new again. Don't for one second think that a vagina can sustain that amount of trauma and not suffer the consequences. In Hubs' words "down there looked like a grizzly bear had attacked". Luckily Hubs had previously delivered calves on farms so wasn't totally scarred for life by seeing, what used to be his favourite place, in tatters.

After I got back to my room, where Hubs and our son were waiting patiently, and the spinal block wore off (thanks again for the timely anaesthetic, guys!), I felt like a grizzly bear had attacked me. I suppose they don't call them third degree tears for nothing. But again, it paled in significance to our new bouncing baby boy. This feeling really was like they describe in the movies. I could not let go of him, and even that night, after Hubs had gone home to get some well-deserved sleep, I cuddled him and took photos of us. I posted a picture of him online, forceps marks and all, and the floodgates of birth and forceps stories opened. I didn't realise how many of my friends' babies had been delivered with forceps. This made me realise that the birth we learn about in antenatal class is as rare as... well, the straight-forward, non-intervention, non-tearing birth we learn about in antenatal class. And I thought, I wish someone had told me that.

Throughout the first few months, after I had my first baby, I noticed two things:

1) New mothers are willing, and eager, to talk about anything and everything related to their birth, no matter how personal, embarrassing or disgusting (in fact they don't even need to know you very well to divulge it all), and

2) That many, many new mums utter the words "I wish someone had told me..." when speaking about their birth and postpartum experiences.

I say mums but really I mean me. I am one of them. I have told stories to strangers that Hubs would die of embarrassment of. Hey, I started this book with the story of my first-born's delivery; completely unprompted. However, in my opinion mums must tell their story. Not only to empower other mothers but because birth stories are like a badge of honour. We are strong, we gave life and we are navigating matrescence like a boss.

I truly hope this book encourages you to share your experience – one unspoken truth at a time.

LABOUR

BEFORE THE FUN BEGINS

I WISH SOMEONE HAD TOLD ME ...
MY BABY WILL COME WHEN IT IS GOOD AND READY

You can try all the tricks in the book (and there are so many!) but if your baby isn't ready to come into the world yet, none of these things will work. I know that your best friend's sister's aunt's old school mate swears by raspberry leaf tea or large amounts of pineapple, even a very hot curry, but the truth is your baby really needs to be teetering on the edge of coming into the world before sex, long walks or membrane sweeps will tip her into your arms. By all means try the methods. Try them all. I did and I still had babies that were seven, eight and nine days late. Babies just come when they are good and ready, I'm afraid.

I WISH SOMEONE HAD TOLD ME ...
I NEED TO PREPARE MYSELF FOR LABOUR

Physically, mentally and emotionally, you need to be ready for this. How you get yourself to that point is up to you (reading this book is a good start!) but when your baby decides it wants to come into the world, you'd better be ready on all fronts. This isn't a last minute decision to duck into the servo for a frozen coke! You are about to give birth to a human!!! It's not called labour for nothing; it is hard work. You really need to give 100% of yourself on all levels. So while you actually don't know what is in store yet, you can prepare yourself. You'll be thankful you did because it'll make it an even more wonderful experience for you.

I WISH SOMEONE HAD TOLD ME ...
THAT I COULD HAVE CONTRACTIONS AND NOT BE IN LABOUR

Yep, totally ripped off! They are called Braxton Hicks contractions and may go on for weeks before your bub arrives. They help your cervix prepare to dilate, so it can move forward and begin shortening and thinning (ripening, softening, effacing... sound familiar?). The good news is that although you can probably feel them they will rarely disrupt what you are doing. For first-timers there's even better news: you will probably have Braxton Hicks contractions without even noticing. With each of these pre-labour contractions your body is preparing to deliver your baby, and if you're really lucky you may find at a check-up that you're already 3cm dilated without having started proper labour.

I WISH SOMEONE HAD TOLD ME …
LOSING MY MUCOUS PLUG OR HAVING A BLOODY SHOW DOES NOT MEAN I AM IN LABOUR

Mucous what? A plug inside me? Losing your mucous plug, which sealed off your cervix during pregnancy (to prevent infection reaching the baby), indicates your cervix is dilating. Sounds gross, is gross! It's described as thick and sticky, either cloudy or clear in colour, sometimes even blood stained (hence the term bloody show). Some women say it looks like a glob of semen or snot! #delicious. Mine looked like solid snot but when I tried to squish it with toilet paper it didn't feel hard. Your plug can also come out in pieces, as mine did. So, it was even harder to decode exactly what was going on there (perhaps it was the beginning of my dignity going down the toilet?). I didn't even see my plug with Baby #1 or #3, but with #2 I noticed my bloody show about two weeks before he came. Sadly, there is no hard and fast rule as to when your baby will come once your plug goes – it can be hours, days or weeks away. Rest assured though that your baby is on the home stretch…

I WISH SOMEONE HAD TOLD ME …
THAT I WILL JUST *KNOW* WHEN I AM IN LABOUR

Like most women, I agonised a lot when I was pregnant with my first: how would I know I was in labour? What if I miss it and then all of a sudden have the baby on the kitchen floor? I know I am not alone in this and will confess that even when I started feeling twinges with my second baby I thought: is this it? I urged Hubs to please go to work a little later that day just to see "if this is going anywhere". Sure enough, about 20 minutes later I told him to call the office because he wasn't coming in; baby was coming out! I just knew that this was *it*. Same with my littlest one who "knocked on my door" for about two weeks before she actually came (nine days late!!!). Yes, she did trick me once or twice but never enough for me to grab my bag and trek to the hospital. When she eventually was ready to meet us, I just knew. And you will too.

I WISH SOMEONE HAD TOLD ME …
THAT I SHOULD TRUST MY INTUITION

Funnily enough, other than just *knowing*, there are other things I observed which indicated to me (in hindsight) that I was in labour. For example, when the twinges with Baby #2 were not even really registering on my pain scale, Hubs was on the phone to a friend who was enquiring if we had the baby yet (YES, we had the baby and just didn't tell anyone!). I shouted from the background "the baby will come today!" I remember really believing that too. It wasn't just some smart comment I made due to my frustration of being eight days past my due date. And our baby did come; about six hours later. This may have been a coincidence but I'm a firm believer that you need to trust your (big, round) gut. Do not discount your intuition when it comes to labour and your baby's imminent arrival. In fact, instinct is the key from here on right through your many years of parenting. There's a reason why the saying goes: "Mother knows best".

I WISH SOMEONE HAD TOLD ME …
THAT PEOPLE PREFER TO TELL YOU THE BAD STUFF

Unfortunately, this is not limited to labour and delivery. People love to tell you their, or someone else's, horror stories. "My daughter's friend's sister had her baby alone on her kitchen floor because she didn't get to the hospital in time. And she lost so much blood she almost died!" (Truth: she had a pretty straightforward birth, the ambulance was there as soon as the baby popped out, and baby and mum were fine. But they won't tell you that.) Why people feel the need to divulge or embellish the bad stuff I will never understand. Maybe to make you feel scared? Maybe to make themselves feel better? Who knows! But you will meet people like this, or you may have some of these "kind" people in your life already. Ignore them! Except for this book, don't ignore it. It is not intended to scare you, it is intended to inform, prepare and empower you. BIG difference!

I WISH SOMEONE HAD TOLD ME ...
TO MAKE A LOOSE PLAN FOR AN IN-CASE-OF-EMERGENCY CAESAREAN

Usually, you will be awake in the event of an emergency C-section, so you should be able to call the shots when your baby is born. But sometimes childbirth is more surprising than we would like. In rare cases you may be put under a general anaesthetic to perform a caesarean if there is no time for an epidural, and it is the safest thing for you and your baby. Make sure you share an "in case of" birth plan with your partner and midwife or obstetrician so they know what your wishes are in case you are knocked out. For example, I don't want anyone but my husband (and hospital staff) to hold the baby until I come to.

I WISH SOMEONE HAD TOLD ME ...
TO KEEP MY HOSPITAL BAG LIGHT

It's not a trip to Bali! However, I still packed clothes that I never would have dreamed of wearing once I had my first baby (and a string bikini!!!). For starters they didn't fit (more about that later) but more importantly they were inconvenient. There are plenty of lists of what to pack on the internet. And remember you're not going to be marooned on an island. If you run out of, or have forgotten, something someone who likes you can bring you things.

I WISH SOMEONE HAD TOLD ME ...
I WILL BE FINE DURING LABOUR

You *will* be fine during labour! There, I told you. And you will be. Labour is like nothing you have ever done before but we are made for it. Our bodies know what to do and you will have amazing staff supporting you. You will get through it. Just remember to breathe and let it all happen naturally…. Oh, and it's totally OK to scream!!!

WATERS!

THAT WATERS CAN BREAK BEFORE YOU ARE IN LABOUR

Unlike in the movies, where waters almost always mean immediate intense labour pains, in the real world sometimes waters can break without labour in sight. It doesn't happen very often, but it did to me with Baby #1. As explained in the intro, I heard a loud *POP!* when I was squatting to place presents under the Christmas tree and then felt some moisture in my panty liner. It was a far cry from the gush they depict in the movies (and which is not very common in reality). So much so that I wasn't even sure if my waters had broken. If you are due or overdue keep an eye out for any excess fluid. Glamorous, huh? Get ready, this is just the beginning of not glamorous.

I WISH SOMEONE HAD TOLD ME ...
THAT I MAY BE UNSURE IF MY WATERS HAD BROKEN

After my waters broke, or at least I thought they had, my midwife told me to put in a maternity pad and ring her when it was full. If it was indeed my waters and I didn't just unintentionally wee myself a little, my pad should slowly fill (with waters). When my pad was soaked to its limit, 10 minutes later, I phoned her back. Now there was no doubt that my waters had indeed broken. However, a friend of mine was induced before her due date because she felt some moisture which didn't completely saturate her maternity pad. She said she will never be sure if her waters actually broke – apparently there is such a thing as hindwaters....

I WISH SOMEONE HAD TOLD ME ...
ABOUT HINDWATERS

Hindwaters are the waters from behind baby's head when it is engaged, as opposed to the fluid trapped in front of baby's head i.e. the forewaters we have all heard about. Hindwaters usually flow after the forewaters but sometimes the amniotic fluid-filled sac, i.e. your bag of waters, can get a small hole in it in hindwater territory and trickle out slowly. This may or may not continue until the forewaters break. You see, the amniotic sac has two layers, so sometimes the small hole behind baby's head can be covered by the second sac layer. This can stop your waters trickling all together until the forewaters break. So, if you think that you felt a trickle it could have been that, or maybe you just pee'd yourself a little (note to self: do pelvic floor exercises!!!). Just having fun. But it is possible so call your hospital if you're unsure.

I WISH SOMEONE HAD TOLD ME …
THAT WATERS BREAKING MEANS A TRIP TO THE HOSPITAL

It's not super urgent but getting to the hospital should be pretty high on your list of priorities (that episode of Sex and the City you've watched 20 times before can wait). Your midwife or obstetrician will want to check you once your waters have broken to make sure your amniotic fluid is clear and the baby is in good shape. If you get the green-light on both, they will probably schedule you in for an induction and send you home. Usually labour will begin on its own soon after, but either way you'll be meeting your baby soon. How exciting!

I WISH SOMEONE HAD TOLD ME …
THAT THE WATERS JUST KEEP COMING

And coming and coming and coming… Amniotic fluid replaces itself constantly. The Hollywood big gush and then it's over is such a myth. Once your waters have broken they'll trickle, leak or gush (if you're in the process of pushing) until your baby is born. Every contraction seems to push out more and it feels very warm. So in all honesty, if you have feeling down below and are not in a bath you will wonder if it's your waters or that other yellow water, namely pee.

INDUCTION

I WISH SOMEONE HAD TOLD ME ...
THERE ARE MANY STAGES TO BEING INDUCED

All my babies came on their own. Albeit pretty late, but when they were ready. I was booked in for an induction with all three of them but I think the threat of that was enough for them to make their way out before I-day (induction day). Anyway, I realise now I never knew exactly what an induction was. I thought they hook you up to some intravenous (i.v.) syntocinon and then you went into labour. Turns out that is usually the last port of call. After you have a membrane stretch and sweep and that doesn't bring labour on, you will probably have some synthetic prostaglandin inserted into your va-jay-jay (gel, tablet or pessary) to ripen your cervix. If that is not enough to bring this baby on its way, you may have your waters broken manually (although this is not always the done thing anymore). If all these methods don't work to kick-start your labour, the final option is the syntocinon i.v. drip I was naively thinking of. This is a synthetic form of the hormone oxytocin which the body produces during labour. It brings on contractions. Induced contractions can be quite severe as the body is not getting a steady increase like it would naturally but hey, at least you are now in labour.

I WISH SOMEONE HAD TOLD ME...
THAT A STRETCH AND SWEEP CAN HURT A LOT

So technically the stretch and sweep manually separates the membranes of your bag of waters from your cervix. This releases prostaglandins (baby-will-come-soon hormones) that will prepare your cervix for baby's arrival and hopefully start labour. Be prepared: it involves a rubber glove and at least one lubed finger. Mothers I have spoken to said it brought on labour for them, but it doesn't always work – it didn't for me with any of my overdue monkeys (babies come when they are ready!). Also, it can hurt a lot depending on who does it. My midwives were amazing, so I found it OK. Probably not something I would do for fun in my lunch-hour but considering what it could potentially do, definitely worth the discomfort. So yes, it is as uncomfortable as it sounds but having said that, you haven't had your baby yet!!! So, while you may think a stretch and sweep is a seven out of ten on your current uncomfortable scale, you'll soon re-scale that after you've given birth. Consider this good practise for clenching your teeth, ummm I mean practising your deep breathing.

I WISH SOMEONE HAD TOLD ME ...
ABOUT THE PAIN OF DRAGGING MY CERVIX FORWARD

I have spoken to quite a few women that say their cervix was manually pulled forward by their midwife or obstetrician as a means to encourage labour. Apparently it is often done during a stretch and sweep to, similarly, speed things up and get Baby moving. But mostly they do this when baby is overdue. So because it is usually done during an S&S (cool acronym alert!) the women who have had their cervix brought forward said that the S&S was a walk in the park in comparison. Sounds awful, doesn't it? And from what I hear…it is Uncomfortable with a capital U!

I WISH SOMEONE HAD TOLD ME ...
THAT BREAKING WATERS MANUALLY CAN HURT

Your midwife may suggest breaking your waters manually to bring labour on or speed things up. For this they use a device that is not too dissimilar to a crochet hook. It is used to nick your amniotic fluid-filled sac i.e. bag of waters. Some women find this painful while others say they didn't notice it much at all. Everyone is different.

I WISH SOMEONE HAD TOLD ME...
THAT A BALLOON CAN RIPEN MY CERVIX

Please don't run to your local shop and buy a bag of party balloons!!!
A Foley's catheter is a *special* balloon used instead of medication to
get the labour show on the road. The catheter has a small uninflated
balloon attached to the end and is inserted into your cervix. There
it is filled with water which puts pressure on your cervix, thereby
releasing prostaglandins. Remember, those are the awesome hormones
that ripen the cervix. When your cervix is open and soft the balloon
falls out. The catheter is then also removed, so don't worry you won't
need to birth that as well. Birthing your baby is definitely enough.

HERE WE GO!

I WISH SOMEONE HAD TOLD ME...
THAT LABOUR COULD BE SO SLOW

Some labours are excruciatingly slow. They can last days! Often these are cheeky first babies. Enjoy the time (as much as you can). Grab your hot water bottle, box set of Sex and the City, some yummy snacks and stand-by, soon your life will change forever (in the most amazing way).

I WISH SOMEONE HAD TOLD ME...
MY BELLY WOULD TAKE ON A STRANGE SHAPE

When your baby is making itself known (*read*: you're definitely in labour) strange things can happen to your baby bump. Generally, the skin on all tummies will tighten extensively but sometimes your belly may change shape. With my first, my bump took on a strange cone shape. The tip of my tummy was much more narrow than the rest, almost like someone had been at it with a ventouse (the suction cup used in some assisted deliveries). Maybe it was a sign of things to come because my eldest, unfortunately, became intimately acquainted with the ventouse during his delivery (and the forceps… but you already know that story).

I WISH SOMEONE HAD TOLD ME…
TO EAT BEFORE I GO TO THE HOSPITAL

The hospital is unlikely to give you food during labour, so if you can stomach it, eat a little at home or bring some light snacks with you. You need all the strength you can get right now because labour, as defined by the Oxford Dictionary = *verb*: work hard; make great effort. Preferably eat foods that give you energy and will help you poo. Apparently, if you poo lots during labour, it'll be less likely you will poo while giving birth. Except that was never the case for me, so good luck with that!

I WISH SOMEONE HAD TOLD ME…
TO HAND IN MY DIGNITY AT THE HOSPITAL DOOR

Where do I start? Is it the fact that all and sundry are going to see your vagina, your bum and probably your boobs? Is it because there will be blood, gunk and probably poo and pee all over the bed, your bath or wherever you choose to have your baby, because you are pushing so hard. Or is it because words will come out of your mouth that are usually reserved for truck drivers? (No offence to our hardworking truckies by the way). Whatever it is, don't be precious. You really do leave your dignity at the door of the hospital when you come in in labour; like a coat check. They should give you a ticket stub for you to collect what's left of it when you are discharged.

I WISH SOMEONE HAD TOLD ME ...
MIDWIVES WOULD GUIDE MY DELIVERY

Where would we be without our amazing midwives? If you are under obstetric care (in Australia this means you have chosen a private hospital), your obstetrician is the woman or man that actually delivers your baby. However, midwives are the ones who will carry you through your labour and delivery experience in a private or public hospital. If you are a private patient, obstetricians have been known to fly through the door just in time to catch the baby as it comes into the world (a role which is massive, don't get me wrong!), but midwives do the rest. If you are a public patient, a midwife will do everything, including delivering your baby. In most circumstances (unless you are birthing through a midwifery group practice) you will meet your midwife only once you arrive at the hospital in labour. By the time you leave you will love them almost as much as your newborn (or at least you will be really, really, really grateful).

I WISH SOMEONE HAD TOLD ME...
THAT "CHECKING MY PROGRESS" COULD BE PAINFUL

The progress check discomfort really varies from woman to woman, and depends on how much your contractions are bothering you at the time and how dilated you are. When you are in a world-of-pain with contractions, a couple of fingers in your 'giney to check the state of your cervix are not going to bother you too much. However, if you've just arrived at the hospital and still have all the fun ahead of you, the cervical check might be a little more on the uncomfortable side.

I WISH SOMEONE HAD TOLD ME...
THAT SMALL HANDS DO NOT MEAN LESS DISCOMFORT

Of course that doesn't mean the size of your hands. No, no, no, the size of your caregiver's hands! Prodding and pushing in your vagina during an examination hurts just as much by someone who wears XS-sized gloves to someone who wears XL ones. That is all!

I WISH SOMEONE HAD TOLD ME...
ABOUT THE VOMITING

I never vomited during labour with my kids but by Kraken did I feel Nauseous. Yes, that's with a capital N!!! Especially with #1. This was one of the reasons I never tried the gas and air. The thought of sticking a plastic mask on my mouth and nose and breathing in that odd smelling vapour was almost enough to make me puke. I am sure the actual thing would have made me hurl. But apparently vomiting is not such a bad thing. It generally signals that things are moving along nicely, and may also aid dilation of the cervix. #SilverLining???

TOO LATE TO BACK OUT NOW

I WISH SOMEONE HAD TOLD ME ...
TO RELAX MY FACE AND REMEMBER TO BREATHE

When my first baby was imminent, a friend of mine gifted me the wonderful saying "loose face, loose fanny!" This might seem a bit odd for our American and Canadian friends, but in Australia fanny is a colloquial term for vagina. Her point: relax! And it's so true. If you scrunch up your face you will likely scrunch up the rest of your body too. The best way to stay relaxed is to breathe. Your breath will be your ally. You will never have appreciated the power of your breath until you use it during labour. It will also come in pretty handy when you have three little ankle-biters fighting, making a mess and crying while you're trying to make dinner (not that my kids ever act in such a manner ☺). I digress. Yep, labour is a good time to become best friends with your breath.

I WISH SOMEONE HAD TOLD ME ...
THAT MOST LABOURS ARE NOT TEXTBOOK

So, you have read all the books, done the courses, watched the videos and bought the t-shirt? Please remember that most labours are <u>not</u> textbook. Be it the timing of contractions, when/how your waters break, what position your baby is in or how quickly your cherub wants to enter the world. Be prepared for anything and remember that the textbook is just that, a textbook. Take the science and general gist from it and leave the rest to intuition. You'll be fine, your body will know what to do!

I WISH SOMEONE HAD TOLD ME ...
THAT SOME PEOPLE DON'T KNOCK WHEN COMING INTO YOUR DELIVERY ROOM

Dignity and embarrassment are on the coat rack? Check! Now add your pride. People will come and go. Some to wish you luck, some to have a peek. Most won't knock, and while this may be the height of rudeness in the beginning, towards the end you won't even notice, or care, anymore.

I WISH SOMEONE HAD TOLD ME ...
I COULD ASK FOR A DIFFERENT MIDWIFE

OK, let's be realistic here, you don't just want to ask for a new midwife because you can. There has to be some serious non-gelling, aka inharmonious energy, going on to make such a big request. After all, you are in labour, how much extra drama do you want to take on? Midwives are the ones who are likely to be there with you from when you come into hospital in labour to when your baby is born. He/she will be your friend, and if he/she is not your friend, you should try to make them your friend. If that doesn't work, you will force them to be your friend and if that still doesn't work, then yes you can request a different midwife. In all likelihood, you will not care as he/she will be the one that finally helps you end the pain by bringing your baby safely into the world. But if you feel uncomfortable or disrespected then by all means exercise that right. Your birthing experience should be wonderful, so everything must fall into place, including your caregiver.

I WISH SOMEONE HAD TOLD ME ...
LABOUR WOULD HURT SO MUCH

Even if you haven't had a baby yet you're probably thinking "Derrrrr, I already knew it hurts!" Well, nobody can blame you for thinking that; it seems to be the first thing women (and men!) learn about the whole process. I don't want to scare you, but no-one can ever *really* prepare you for how much it will hurt. If you are pregnant with your first baby, (or just need a refresher, if you're having more babies) *this* is the truth. The pain of labour is like nothing else. If you choose to go the "natural" route without gas/air and drugs, you will probably wonder how you survived it. After my first was born I remember thinking about how much it would hurt to have your fingernails pulled out with tweezers. Surely it could not hurt as much as labour. Of course it doesn't start off like that; your body is smart and eases you into it. It gives your brain a chance to send some lovely beta-endorphins (a peptide which naturally activates pain relief) around your system to try to deal with what is happening. No matter how long or short your labour is, there will probably come a point when you think you can't endure any more pain, but you can and you will! And then you are holding your new baby in your arms, and tears of pain are replaced with tears of joy. It may not be that day, but soon you will forget how much it hurt and you will probably want to do it all over again. #SoWorthIt

I WISH SOMEONE HAD TOLD ME…
LABOUR MAY BE JUST AS PAINFUL WITH SUBSEQUENT BABIES

Oh yes, labour hurts regardless of whether it's your first baby or your 15th. OK, I haven't had 15 babies, so please correct me if I am wrong, but I have had three, and they were all excruciating in their own special way ☺.

I WISH SOMEONE HAD TOLD ME ...
THAT I WOULD GET SO THIRSTY DURING LABOUR

All that huffing, puffing, grunting, and in my case screaming, sure dries out your mouth and throat. Have some water in your hospital bag that you can sip on throughout. A wet whistle will not only minimise discomfort but also keep you hydrated in case you have a long journey ahead.

I WISH SOMEONE HAD TOLD ME ...
THAT MY BODY WILL RELIEVE THE PAIN

OK, so it's not like having an epidural, but your body is designed to deliver babies and therefore knows what it needs to do. In terms of pain relief, we have sweet neurotransmitters (fancy word for messengers) called beta-endorphins within us that make the whole ride a little less painful. Beta-endorphins activate our opioid receptors thereby dulling the pain. This process has a similar effect as opioid drugs, such as morphine and pethidine, but on a natural, less intense level. Your body is brilliant. If you can, try really hard to switch off your mind and trust your body!

BABY IS COMING

I PROBABLY WON'T STICK TO MY BIRTH PLAN

Ah yes, the birth plan. By all means write one. Analyse it, discuss it with your birth partner and your midwife and/or obstetrician. Learn it by heart and visualise it. Then throw it away! While it is a great idea to have a birth plan, it is best to use it only as a guide. So much can happen during labour that you have no control over. If you are strict on what you would like to happen you may feel disappointed when your plan goes off-course. Please don't let your hopes of a "perfect birth" ruin what will irrespectively be one of, if not *the* most amazing day of your life. Having said that, any aspects of your birth that you do have control over, such as what injections your newborn shall receive and an in-case-of-caesarean plan, are a good idea to discuss with your caregiver in detail beforehand. You may not be in a state where you feel you can make these decisions when/if it comes to the crunch.

I WISH SOMEONE HAD TOLD ME ...
THAT I WOULD FORGET MOST THINGS I LEARNT FROM THE BOOKS AND BIRTHING CLASSES ONCE IN REAL LABOUR

I kind of remembered that if they press the red button on the wall you're in strife! So, I don't think that we forget everything. But in all honesty a lot of what you learn will be forgotten when you are in true labour. Please do read it all though; something will stick. Just don't think that you will be able to follow everything to a T once your baby takes over and your brain clocks off.

I WISH SOMEONE HAD TOLD ME ...
I WOULD GET ANNOYED WITH PEOPLE IN MY HOSPITAL ROOM

This is not just reserved for your partner, but anyone else that is present too. With my first baby, I snarled at the student midwife who was rubbing my back (she mysteriously disappeared out of the room soon after never to return. Sorry!!!! If you are reading this, I hope you can forgive me). She was just trying to comfort me, I know, but it was so annoying. I had no tolerance for it. I have also heard of women who hurled abuse at their midwife or obstetrician because they were telling them to push. There is no shortage of things women get annoyed about when in labour. You'll understand when you are in the situation. It is honestly not malicious. We'll just call it primal! #PottyMouth

I WISH SOMEONE HAD TOLD ME …
THAT CERVICAL DILATION CAN DECREASE DURING LABOUR

OK, I really hadn't heard about this before researching this book but when a couple of mums mentioned this had happened to them I became intrigued. My first quick research brought up only information that this phenomenon is absurd. The likely explanation was that different midwives had done the dilation check and therefore there was a discrepancy, or that the person who checked the cervix was inexperienced. Then I came across a journal article by Ina May Gaskin, the widely renowned "mother of authentic midwifery". She describes this phenomenon called Pasmo[1]: when women are frightened, full of adrenalin or overwhelmed the cervix can sometimes slightly close again. The idea is that women then have a chance to get into a situation where they feel safer and more comfortable to give birth. Take home message: remain as calm as you can. Being told you have gone backwards in dilation must be unbearable.

I WISH SOMEONE HAD TOLD ME …
THAT SOONER OR LATER I WON'T CARE HOW MANY PEOPLE SEE MY BOOBS, BUM AND VAGINA

I have a friend who has a birth mark on her bum (you know who you are!). She hates this birth mark more than anything else about herself. So when she was pregnant she wanted it to be known that no-one shall, under any circumstances, see her bottom while she is giving birth. Fast forward into 12 hours of hard labour and she is on all-fours with her bum in the air, while wearing only a back-gaping hospital gown! Me on the other hand, I packed a bikini top in my hospital bag with #1 (note to self: *not* packing for Bali) because I didn't want anyone to see my boobs while I had a water birth. Like my friend, by the time I was 9cm dilated I would have streaked the whole hospital completely naked, if it would have made the pain subside. In short, you just don't care in the late stages of labour; it takes over. Remember your dignity, embarrassment and pride are waiting for you at the hospital door.

I WISH SOMEONE HAD TOLD ME ...
THAT EACH LABOUR WILL BE DIFFERENT

Never mind the labour from one woman to another, subsequent labours of one mother can be completely different too. I had three very different labours with my three kids. With my first my waters broke 11 hours before my first contraction. I found his labour to be quite bearable (well, as bearable as labour can be). My second was super quick and super intense. He didn't let us know he was coming until he was almost already here. My waters broke about halfway between first contraction and baby being born. All too fast. Quite unbearable! My third told me she was on the way for about two weeks before she came. I had severe Braxton Hicks and on more than one occasion phoned Hubs to put him on "notice" but she never came! Her labour was great (if you're into pain and stuff!). Textbook. Totally bearable. Waters broke while pushing.

Each labour was so unique, like they are now as children; all painful in their own way ☺.

I WISH SOMEONE HAD TOLD ME ...
THAT LABOUR COULD BE SO QUICK

Generally subsequent babies will come quicker but sometimes the first one can make a speedy entrance too. All I can say is: Be Prepared! I know of women who dilated from 3cm to 10cm in 40 minutes with nothing more than red cheeks (bum and face ☺)! It happens.

I WISH SOMEONE HAD TOLD ME ...
THAT A QUICKER LABOUR IS NOT NECESSARILY
AN EASIER LABOUR

All the same stuff needs to happen to get your baby out; it just happens at a faster rate. I personally found it harder, the quicker my labours were. Less time to "get in the zone" (or no time if it's all happening *really* quickly), and all my pain was squeezed into a shorter space of time. On the other hand, it was over quicker and I felt I recovered better and more rapidly. But that was just my experience. Some women I have spoken to found their quicker labours easier, and some found the speed of the labour made no difference to their birthing experience.

I WISH SOMEONE HAD TOLD ME ...
I WOULD DILATE SO QUICKLY THAT THERE WAS NO TIME FOR DRUGS

There is a cut-off point for pain relief. It is for the safety of you and your baby. If you really want something to "take the edge off" don't stay at home too long when labouring, and make sure you discuss pain relief with your midwife or obstetrician before you go into labour. They can give you a better indication about what you can have, when, and what point is considered too late.

I WISH SOMEONE HAD TOLD ME ...
THAT THE POSITION OR ANGLE OF THE BABY COMING DOWN THE BIRTH CANAL COULD CAUSE ME SUCH MISERY

We've all heard of babies lying in a breech position (head up, rather than down), which can make birth a little tricky. But there are other positions and angles that could make it all a bit more agonising too. For instance, when both my boys came down the birth canal (head first, mind you!) the place I felt it most was in my hips, more specifically in my hip joints. When I pushed to get them out it felt like some strong men were pulling my legs and trying to dislocate my hip joints. I still remember it vividly. Oh so painful! Another mother told me her baby pushed on her bladder in such a way that she could not pee. She had to have a catheter inserted just so she could empty her bladder! Other babies' positions and angles can pinch nerves, cause twitches or really just hurt like crazy.

I WISH SOMEONE HAD TOLD ME ...
THAT YOU CAN HAVE A HIP LABOUR

I personally wish someone had told me this, but when researching this book, I found that it is actually quite uncommon and quite possible that no-one I know has ever gone through it.

I had hip labours with both my boys (#1 and #2) and it was the worst thing. The only way I can describe it is like someone is pulling on your leg trying to pull your hip out of its ball-and-socket joint. Both hips, at the same time, during every contraction, especially when pushing. The pain for me was so intense that I cannot remember feeling the actual contractions at that point. Nor did I feel my babies move down the birth canal. All I felt was like I was in a torture hold where one contraption was trying to dislocate my right hip and another one my left.

When I had my first baby I thought this was just because he was so big and I also had forceps in there creating more pressure. But when I also felt it with my second boy, who was a bit smaller and the birth was a very straightforward water birth, my midwife told me it must be just the way I am put together. OUCH! You can imagine I was already scared about birthing my third baby before she was even conceived.

However, now knowing that the pain is probably specific to my body, I did everything possible to prevent the hip pain with #3. I attended pregnancy Pilates regularly, I walked a lot, I got pregnancy massages by a professional remedial massage therapist who focused on the muscles around my hips, and I saw a women's health physiotherapist who treated me regularly to help loosen up the area. I know it sounds like a lot, but it was worth it because it worked! My baby girl (#3) was born with only the most minimal (*read*: normal) hip discomfort. She did come out with her head turned to the side so that wasn't super pleasant but ridiculous hip pain? Nope. None.

I WISH SOMEONE HAD TOLD ME ...
I COULD HAVE AN ORGASM DURING LABOUR

No way!?! It's true, I swear. Apparently 0.3% of women experience orgasmic waves while giving birth[2]. So imagine, while you're moaning and groaning through a contraction, it suddenly turns into moaning and groaning of a different kind. I think this is awesome on so many levels. The scientist in me is having an orgasm just thinking about this amazingness. A mother I met told me about her orgasmic birth experience. She said it was actually more embarrassing than pleasurable for her because she didn't expect it. However, there are women out there that use sexual stimulation as a form of pain relief. Well, whatever gets you through, I say.

I WISH SOMEONE HAD TOLD ME ...
THAT I WILL GET TO A POINT WHERE I REALLY THINK I CAN'T GO ON ANYMORE

Some women have told me that they started packing their bags to leave the hospital. Others said they were trying to walk out the door in next to no clothes. I don't think I did any of those things (I'll have to check with Hubs) but I do remember saying, all three times, "I can't do this anymore". I'm certain I didn't just say it because I didn't want to do it anymore, I was positive I couldn't do it anymore. "I can't do it anymore" and its variations, are music to a midwife's ears because it indicates you are in transition i.e. almost at the finish line. Provided everything goes smoothly, your baby will be here very, very soon.

I WISH SOMEONE HAD TOLD ME ...
TO DO WHATEVER GETS ME THROUGH

OK, so I think we've established that labour is pretty painful for most women. You will likely be in a zone like no other and you will do whatever it takes to get you through. For some this is screaming the hospital down, while others manage their pain with a vibrator (no, not a typo, I meant to write vibrator). Whatever it is, when you're at that point, and you will know what point I'm talking about when you get there, you should do whatever feels right at the time, no matter who is watching. Don't feel embarrassed! And if you need reassurance that your reaction is normal, watch an episode of *One Born Every Minute*.

PAIN RELIEF

TO MAKE MY INTENTIONS ABOUT AN EPIDURAL VERY CLEAR

If there is even the tiniest chance that you may want an epidural, make sure you tell someone in your corner when you get to the hospital, i.e. a midwife or someone else who can sort that out for you. There are a very limited number of anaesthetists around the hospital and you want your name on their list as soon as you require an epidural. Apparently, unless there is a complication, epidurals are given on a first-in, best-dressed basis. What an analogy when you are likely to be naked or scantily-clad when that epidural is administered.

I WISH SOMEONE HAD TOLD ME ...
IT'S OK TO CHANGE MY MIND ABOUT THE DRUGS

Your loose birth plan should include loose intentions about pain relief during labour. You may go in wanting a completely natural and drug-free birth but then things take an unexpected turn. You could end up being in labour much longer than anticipated or the pain just becomes too much. Nobody will judge you if you change your mind. And nor should you judge yourself. It. Is. OK!

I WISH SOMEONE HAD TOLD ME ...
THAT EPIDURALS ARE NOT ALWAYS 100% EFFECTIVE

Yes, sometimes the epidural does not do the whole job. The needle needs to be placed in your spine with pin-point (no pun intended!) accuracy to get the full effect. The doctors that give you the epidural are professionals so will most likely hit a bullseye first time, meaning sweet, sweet pain relief is on its way. But sometimes it doesn't work out that way, especially if the mum's a squirmer ☺.

I WISH SOMEONE HAD TOLD ME ...
THAT MY EPIDURAL MIGHT NEED TO BE RE-INSERTED

If your epidural has not been placed in exactly the right spot the two most likely consequences are:

1) You feel no or very little pain relief, and/or

2) The placement of your epidural pinches a nerve.

The first is annoying because the drugs aren't kicking in… yet. Whereas the second can be really uncomfortable but also funny. One mum told me the twinging of the nerve made her leg kick involuntarily, kicking her partner right in the belly. Either way, your epidural may need to be re-inserted to a more suitable position. Take a breath, don't get frustrated and whatever you do, don't move!

I WISH SOMEONE HAD TOLD ME…
THAT HAVING AN EPIDURAL INSERTED IS NOT THAT BAD

I guess it depends on who you speak to, what situation you are in and what you are expecting (and consider bad). Unless you are getting "prepped" for a scheduled caesarean, you will usually be in sufficient pain by the time you have your epidural, that the discomfort of the insertion will leave you unfazed. You will probably feel relieved knowing the pain will subside soon. And let's face it, a small needle in your back is nothing compared to pushing a watermelon out of your lady garden, is it?

I WISH SOMEONE HAD TOLD ME …
I WOULD SHAKE UNCONTROLLABLY WHEN I HAVE AN EPIDURAL

You probably already know that spinal pain relief, such as an epidural or a spinal block, can have some side effects. Ones I hear about often are shaking, feeling cold and even teeth chattering. The exact reason behind this is unknown. But while it is more common in mothers who have had an epidural, shaking can also happen when a mum has had no pain relief. So interesting! Mums who have experienced shaking due to their epidural say it is quite unpleasant and can be so severe you can't speak properly or may be too afraid to hold your new baby. One mum told me she was so scared to hold her daughter when she was born, she feared she may drop her. Poor mummy! Luckily the shaking and other side effects will wear off. Best to chat with your midwife or obstetrician before you go into labour to get the low-down on pain relief so you're informed if/when the time comes.

I WISH SOMEONE HAD TOLD ME …
THAT I WILL NEED A URINARY CATHETER INSERTED IF I HAVE AN EPIDURAL

Unless you want to continuously pee yourself until your epidural has worn off, it's best to get a urinary catheter inserted (jokes of course, you don't have a choice. Epidural = catheter). The epidural will dampen the sensation of you needing to pee and your legs will probably be too numb to walk to the loo anyway, so a urinary catheter will be inserted once your epidural has taken effect. This shouldn't hurt, as your epidural is nicely numbing you from about the belly button down. But it could be slightly uncomfortable when it is removed after you've had the baby, as the epidural will have worn off. Although pain is all relative really, isn't it? You've just had a baby, once your epidural wears off the removal of the catheter will probably be one of your lesser worries.

I WISH SOMEONE HAD TOLD ME...
THAT THE DRUGS AND/OR GAS AND AIR COULD MAKE ME FEEL SO NAUSEOUS

Unfortunately, nausea from pain relief is a common side effect. Make sure you discuss this with your obstetrician or midwife when you talk about pain relief, especially if you are as spew-averse as me. Mind you, labour can be so nauseating in its own right. Many women vomit before, during and after giving birth, drugs or no drugs. Yippee!!!!

DELIVERY AND IMMEDIATELY AFTER

WE'RE ON!

GIVING BIRTH IS NOTHING LIKE IN THE MOVIES

Yes, let's just throw that myth out right from the start. Hollywood lies! There is so much more to it than pant...scream...swear...push... baby! The image of Rachel in *Friends* having her baby comes to mind. Her make-up is immaculate; her hair is in gorgeous pigtails. She has a little sweat on her brow and, although she is apparently in a lot of pain, she is totally lucid making smart comments to everyone including the obstetrician. If you have that image of childbirth in your mind's eye, please wipe it now. That's not what happens in real life. Real childbirth is so much more... let's call it *juicy*.

I WISH SOMEONE HAD TOLD ME ...
THAT THE BOOKS AND VIDEOS SUGAR-COAT IT ALL

The books, videos, classes etc. will help teach you a lot about childbirth, but nothing can ever *really* prepare you for giving birth. You just need to do it. Within the hour of having our first boy Hubs said to me "they didn't show that in any of the videos". And he's right. The videos we saw showed a lighter side of childbirth (understatement of the year!), a birthing process which some women may experience but, realistically, so many don't. Unfortunately, I do not think they would get away with saying:

- It hurts *so* much more than you could ever imagine

- Things can go wrong, aka off-the-birth-plan-rails

- If it's your first baby your odds of needing a little help (i.e. "intervention" in medical speak) to get the baby out (such as ventouse or forceps, which may come with the dreaded episiotomy) are quite high; and

- Babies are demanding from day one (yup, definitely not like getting a puppy)

Mmm, wonder if *I* can get away with saying all this?

I WISH SOMEONE HAD TOLD ME ...
TO IGNORE THE BOOKS AND GO WITH WHAT I FEEL (EXCEPT FOR THIS BOOK, OF COURSE ☺)

Many mums have told me something to this effect. And while there are some amazing birth guides on the market, every woman's birth is so different. A book or course can't possibly cover all the scenarios. Sure there is one common outcome but the road to this is not nearly as clear-cut. The bottom line is: trust your instincts. Only you know what you are feeling, and this will instinctively lead you to what it is you need to do. We are animals and never more so than when our primal instincts take over while giving birth. Be primal, baby! Scream, grunt, moan, move or do whatever it is that you feel you need to do. And if you feel you need to push, then it is probably time to push. Luckily, we have our wonderful midwives and obstetricians by our side to guide us through, but you are the only one who can *feel* what's next. Trust your gut!

I WISH SOMEONE HAD TOLD ME ...
THAT I MAY VOMIT – BEFORE, DURING AND AFTER GIVING BIRTH

While it is quite common for women to vomit during the first stage of labour, occasionally a poor mother-to-be may vomit throughout the whole process (like the actual "labour" of childbirth isn't enough already!). Just like some women have morning/all-day sickness for their entire pregnancy, it is so hard to predict whatchyagonnaget. The physical cause of the continued vomiting is not really known, other than that the woman may be overexerted or possibly reacting to opiates, such as pethidine, given for pain relief. I did feel incredibly nauseous during my first labour and consciously chose not to use gas and air because of fear it may actually make me vomit. The thought of vomiting once was too much for me to bear, I can't imagine how the poor ladies cope who vomit throughout.

I WISH SOMEONE HAD TOLD ME ...
THAT I MAY HAVE TO WALK TO GET THE BABY'S HEAD INTO THE RIGHT POSITION

Walking is one of the best ways to position the baby's head to get him ready to pop out (oh, if only it was as easy as "pop!"). Walking is not exclusive to early labour. I have heard of women walking the corridors of the hospital after already labouring for many hours, to help get the head in the right spot. It is rare, because more often than not by that stage the head is already in a favourable position, but it can happen. So, I thought I better put a little section in here, just so everyone else can know it too. You know, just in case...

I WISH SOMEONE HAD TOLD ME ...
I AM PROBABLY NOT AS FUNNY AS I THINK WHILE ON MORPHINE

Pain relief is goooooood, there are no two ways about it. If you can tolerate it, morphine is especially good, and also makes light of a painful situation. It can also make you a bit light-headed (it's a narcotic after all) and happy. I have spoken to lots of women who told me they thought they were Billy Connolly while on morphine; telling hilarious jokes to all people present (even if they have just met them). On reflection, they told me, they didn't think people were actually laughing *at* their jokes (but I'm sure they got a giggle anyway).

I WISH SOMEONE HAD TOLD ME ...
HOW MUCH I WOULD ITCH FROM PAIN MEDICINE

Unfortunately, itching is a common and unpleasant side effect of some drugs, including opioids, such as fentanyl, morphine and pethidine. Whichever way you receive your pain meds, epidural, spinal block or injection, the itching can be really unpleasant (fits with the theme of childbirth, doesn't it? ☺) and annoying. Put your partner on scratching duty...

Luckily, the itching should be pretty short-lived – once your baby is here, your itch will soon disappear (sorry, clearly I am not a poet in my spare time).

I WISH SOMEONE HAD TOLD ME ...
THAT I MAY GET SO TIRED I WILL FORGET EVERYTHING I LEARNT

Or you may just forget the stuff you learnt because your mind is focused on pushing an approximate 3kg baby out of your va-jay-jay. Either way, rest assured (rest ha, ha, yeah right!) your body knows what to do. It really does. You have the knowledge from your books and courses stored in there somewhere but sometimes a woman will get to a point of tiredness, exhaustion and frazzledness during labour where she forgets even the most basic things. And yes, I mean things like your husband's name (it does happen!). Towards the end of my first birth, I literally passed out between contractions and was so rudely awoken when a new contraction began. I was so, so, so tired, there was no way I was remembering stuff I had learnt about childbirth. You just don't know what lies ahead so remember to breathe and trust your big, round gut rather than your head when it comes to the big event. Your body will know what to do

I WISH SOMEONE HAD TOLD ME ...
I WOULD BE FINE

My mum has told me on several occasions that she honestly thought she was dying while giving birth to me (her first baby). She said surely if it hurt that much and was so incredibly intense, someone would have said something to her beforehand. Or at least they should have mentioned that she would get through it in one piece and be fine. Poor Mum! I wish someone had written a book like this before she went through it for the first time. The take home message: it is painful and intense, but you will get through it and you will be fine.

PUSHING

TO ONLY PUSH DURING CONTRACTIONS

Contractions are your body's natural way to help deliver your baby. Your pushing is added support. Although you will probably feel like you have to push (or maybe it'll just feel like you need to do the world's biggest poo!), you should only push during a contraction. When you're in the thick of it, it may seem like ages between contractions, but don't be tempted to push in between unless somebody, who knows what they are doing, tells you to. Use the time between contractions to recover. And remember to breathe!

I WISH SOMEONE HAD TOLD ME...
THAT I MAY NOT BE ALLOWED TO PUSH EVEN IF I FEEL LIKE IT

This is the worst! Well OK, not really the worst, but it's pretty bad... Imagine busting for a pee and you're not allowed to let it out. You feel like you're going to explode, right? Well, it's kinda like that but worse. Your caregiver always has legitimate reasons for denying you a push, of course. Like your cervix hasn't dilated enough yet or that full-on pushing may actually tear your vagina (some more?!?!). But that doesn't take away from the fact that all you want to do is push, push, push. Breathe and try to resist the urge with positive self-talk, such as "my vagina will remain pretty if I don't push right now" or more seriously "it is best for me and my baby if I don't push right now".

I WISH SOMEONE HAD TOLD ME...
THAT PUSHING WILL HURT TOO

You think you are at the tail end of it all and then you get sprung with the pain of pushing. So. Not. Fair! It can be excruciating for some women for many reasons, including it can take a long time, and there may be a spot where you particularly feel it. I felt every shift of my first two babies in my poor, poor hips. I won't bore you again with the details, but pushing was by far the worst part of labour for me when I had my boys. Some women have told me that during the final pushing stages they lost all control of their legs, or even their whole body, and shook involuntarily. On the other hand, some women have told me they found pushing the easiest part. Lucky them!

I WISH SOMEONE HAD TOLD ME ...
THAT PUSHING WOULD BE THE BEST PART OF MY LABOUR

For some women bearing down is like a release and/or relief. With my third it certainly was. The physical act of pushing felt somewhat nice (don't shoot me! I mean nice in the most non-nice way). It is sort of like if you have pent up anger and then finally scream (or go for a run!). Or let's be honest, like when you have PMS and your period finally comes. Aaaah the relief!

I WISH SOMEONE HAD TOLD ME ...
THAT MY BABY SLIPS BACK UP AGAIN AFTER EVERY PUSH

Yeah, because pushing out a baby isn't enough "labour"... Unfortunately, when pushing your baby through your pelvis, the little troublemaker slips back up a little between contractions. Luckily, they don't slip back much but still, think two steps forward, one step back (especially for first-timers). Don't fret though, this is very normal and quite okay as long your baby keeps moving towards the finish-line with each push. You may or may not feel your baby slipping back but rest assured that once you (well not literally you, of course) can see your baby's head you will soon be holding your gorgeous scrunched-up wonder in your arms.

I WISH SOMEONE HAD TOLD ME ...
I MAY NEED TO PUSH FOR A REALLY LONG TIME

The average time spent pushing with your first child is about an hour. Having said that it can be much quicker, or much sloooower. Two hours pushing for your first baby is not uncommon![3] When you're doing it, it seems like forever but luckily you only push during contractions so there is some time in between to catch your breath, relax a little, and remember what you are doing – pushing to meet your baby.

I WISH SOMEONE HAD TOLD ME ...
THAT POSTERIOR BABIES TAKE LONGER TO PUSH OUT

Generally, babies in a posterior position do take a little more 'oomph' to come into the world. Yes, unfortunately more labour in labour. The position of baby's back facing your back means baby is usually not as streamlined for his/her journey through the birth canal. This results in a need to push longer in order to guide your little one through. Unfortunately, this often comes with more pain too due to bub's positioning. I haven't had a posterior baby, i.e. back labour, but women who have asked me to pass on this piece of advice: have an epidural!

I WISH SOMEONE HAD TOLD ME ...
ABOUT THE "RING OF FIRE"

Be honest, who just sang that Johnny Cash song in their head when reading this heading?

I digress. Let's come back to the "ring of fire" in question here... When giving birth, you are pushing a head of about 35cm circumference out of your vagina. You are expanding your vagina to its maximum. Stretching such thin and fragile skin so wide results in a rather unpleasant burning sensation (I can't put it any nicer than that), hence the "ring of fire". Luckily our wonderfully designed bodies know how to combat even this: the burning won't last too long as your max-stretched skin will block the nerve endings in your va-jay-jay, meaning no more pain[4]. The bath is a great place to be at this point. I found it managed to extinguish the fire somewhat, compared to letting that ring burn in the open air.

I WISH SOMEONE HAD TOLD ME ...
I MAY NEED AN EPISIOTOMY

Episi-what-tomy? It's described as a small snip in the woman's perineum (the area between hole one and hole two, down there) but how *small* it actually is, I am not sure. I guess it varies from woman to woman. Episiotomies are rare these days but if you have a stubborn bub, like my first one whose shoulders even got stuck once his head was delivered, the scissors will come out and help make the exit a little larger! It's scary to read, I know, but it is only done if necessary. In the scheme of things it doesn't actually hurt, as they will give you a little local anaesthetic in the area before snipping away. And trust me if you need one it will be at the point where you would do anything to get that tenacious little rascal out of you.

I WISH SOMEONE HAD TOLD ME …
THAT I WILL STILL NEED TO PUSH WHEN MY DOCTOR IS USING THE VENTOUSE OR FORCEPS

The ventouse (suction cup) or forceps are usually pulled out from their secret hiding place when your stubborn munchkin is not coming out on their own, or is getting distressed during the pushing phase. They are designed to give your little one a little help by assisting a little bit. Unfortunately, there is only so much they can do so you will need to push just as much during contractions. There really is no easy way out of childbirth, not even a little bit.

I WISH SOMEONE HAD TOLD ME …
ABOUT FUNDAL PRESSURE

In some instances, when you are pushing your baby out your caregiver may assist by pushing the upper part of your uterus (aka the top part of the human in your tummy) down towards the birth canal (aka the exit) – this is called applying fundal pressure. It is thought to help push the baby in the right direction, basically giving you a helping hand. However, it is a bit controversial as it may lead to a greater chance of tearing, especially the anal sphincter (ouch, yes that's your bum hole!). It is usually only done when the mother has had an epidural and for some women it is apparently really uncomfortable. It's rare these days especially for vaginal births, so you can exhale now. But just in case, don't say I didn't warn you.

I WISH SOMEONE HAD TOLD ME ...
THAT MOST WOMEN POO WHEN PUSHING OUT THEIR BABY

It's our worst nightmare, right? And we all think it won't happen to us, but the truth is it will happen to most of us (even if only a little bit). Poo, number two, faeces, brownie, doodoo, crap or whatever you choose to call it, can and probably will, happen. After all, you are pushing an approximate 3kg mass out of your vagina. You can't push that hard and dictate which hole something will come out of. Unfortunately, in this case sh★t really does happen!

I WISH SOMEONE HAD TOLD ME ...
I COULD FRACTURE OR DISLOCATE MY TAILBONE WHILE GIVING BIRTH

Fractures and dislocations are pretty rare but bruising isn't. As your baby makes its way out, i.e. through the birth canal, there is a lot of pressure being placed on your coccyx, aka tailbone. Ouch!!!

Do I need to say more? My first baby really bruised that area of mine and it was excruciating to sit on for a few weeks. However, a friend of mine had her coccyx actually fractured by her darling son (wowsers!!!) and I have heard of tailbone dislocations too. I can only imagine how that must feel. So now not only are you trying to mend and heal your front bottom, but you will also have to focus some of that healing energy on your real bottom too. If this happens to you, stock up on ice packs, you will need them – one pack for the front and one for the back.

I WISH SOMEONE HAD TOLD ME ...
THAT THE PLACENTA NEEDS TO BE PUSHED OUT TOO

So, you have pushed and pushed and pushed and are finally holding your baby in your arms. And that's enough now, right? No, no, now it's time to deliver the placenta. Known as the third stage of labour, delivering the placenta will happen at different times for different women. Yes, more pushing and more contractions. Although I found the contractions and the actual birthing of the placenta quite bearable, some women have told me that they find these contractions and this pushing phase really full-on. We are all so different! If you had a complicated birth your caregiver may suggest an actively managed third stage (you can also choose this option, if you want) where you are given an injection of syntocinon and the placenta comes away quicker and is removed (*read*: pulled out of you by the cord) by your caregiver. Sounds worse (and grosser) than it is. Or maybe not, it's pretty gross. But you will probably have your bare baby lying on your bare chest at this stage, so the reminder why you need to do this is right there (and oh so worth it!).

I WISH SOMEONE HAD TOLD ME ...
THAT MY PLACENTA MAY NEED TO BE MANUALLY REMOVED

On occasion, but really very rarely, the placenta does not come away from the uterine wall on its own, or it only partially comes away. This can happen even if you have had the syntocinon injection. Unfortunately, this can lead to haemorrhaging and, not to scare you, but haemorrhaging is a leading cause of death for the mother during childbirth. But enough of the doom and gloom, we're having a baby here! So to make sure your retained placenta is finally fully evicted, your placenta will be removed manually (yes, by that I mean by hand!!! Literally). If there is time, and you haven't received one already, you'll get a spinal block or epidural to manage the pain, and some intravenous antibiotics to avoid infection. If you haven't done a pee you may also get a catheter inserted and then it's all systems go. If there isn't time for pain relief, I have heard the removal is extremely painful (maybe that is because you have a grown persons' hand up your honey pot?). But luckily retained placentas are quite uncommon so hopefully this paragraph is the only time you will come across one.

CAESAREAN DELIVERIES

HOW QUICK A CAESAREAN IS

In an emergency, once your obstetrician decides you need a C-section because labour is not progressing, your baby is distressed, or another reason, the time until you meet your baby suddenly comes around very, very quickly. They don't call it emergency for fun (not that any part of having a C-section is "fun"). The time from incision to delivery is usually less than five minutes! Bang, bang!!! No mucking around there. If you are having a scheduled caesarean it will take a bit longer, about 10 to 15 minutes, but it's still very quick in the scheme of things. These times of course don't take into consideration anaesthetics and the delivery of the placenta etc. but you must agree, super quick nonetheless.

I WISH SOMEONE HAD TOLD ME ...
THAT "GETTING THE BABY OUT" DURING A CAESAREAN WOULD BE SO UNCOMFORTABLE

I haven't had a caesarean so I can't speak for myself but I have heard from some mothers that yes, it can be quite uncomfortable when baby gets evicted. Some mums say that when the doctors push on their tummy, during the procedure, it feels like they might explode. Others say they hardly felt a thing. I've also been told that if you have an epidural getting the baby out feels more like a tugging sensation, whereas if you have a spinal block it may feel more like pressure. If you are not ready for it, either can give you quite a shock as it is a sensation you probably haven't felt before. On the flip side, I have spoken to women who said they didn't feel anything, regardless of epidural or spinal. And hey, even if you do, look at the prize you get for your discomfort.

I WISH SOMEONE HAD TOLD ME ...
I MAY NEED A GENERAL ANAESTHETIC

If things become dire quickly or your baby is distressed and your labour is not progressing, your caregiver may opt for a general anaesthetic as a last resort. Yep, that's the one where they knock you out completely. It is very uncommon and of course everything will be done to avoid it, but sometimes it is just necessary, as it is the best thing for you and your baby. That's why I can't stress enough to make the main aim of your birth plan: get the baby out safely (oh, and keep an eye on mum while they're at it)!

I WISH SOMEONE HAD TOLD ME ...
I COULD STILL HAVE A FORCEPS DELIVERY EVEN IF I HAVE A CAESAREAN

Sometimes when a baby is in an unfavourable position, for example tucked in under the ribs (aka not deep in the birth canal), your obstetrician will use forceps or ventouse to deliver your baby via C-section. This can happen even if you are booked in for an elective caesarean. In fact, it happens more often than we realise. For some reason many people think that a caesarean is like a short cut to the baby and that it can just be lifted out as soon as the incision is made. On the contrary, the incision of a C-section is often very small and if the baby is not fully engaged (in the correct position) an assisted caesarean delivery is called for.

I WISH SOMEONE HAD TOLD ME ...
THAT AFTER THE CAESAREAN I WOULD FEEL LIKE I HAD BEEN HIT BY A TRUCK

Again, this will vary from woman to woman. Some women say that having a C-section made them feel soooo terrible that they wanted to stick the baby back in and go out to lunch rather than feel the way they did post-surgery. Whereas some women said they really could go out to lunch after having a caesarean. You can't predict how you will feel, so maybe expect the worst and hope for the best on this one.

I WISH SOMEONE HAD TOLD ME …
I MAY FEEL LIKE A FAILURE AFTER HAVING A CAESAREAN

Remember in the Labour chapter I encouraged you not to write a rigid birth plan. Having a firm plan in place is likely to end in disappointment because babies just do whatever they want, when they want. This is not specific to caesareans, but I know that there are many mothers that felt like failures after they needed a caesarean. Or they feel like they missed out, or let people, including the baby, down. The way you feel is the way you feel, nobody should ever tell you otherwise. Hormones are a bitch, we all know that, and coupled with the disappointment of what you expected, it is understandable you will feel a lot of things. Hopefully you will get through this time quickly by talking to family, friends and experts (if needed), because there is a brand new baby for you to enjoy. To avoid disappointment all together, throw your birth plan in the bin or keep it to one sentence (not judging, just suggesting):

<u>Birth plan</u>

Bring baby safely into the world (however that may be)

I WISH SOMEONE HAD TOLD ME …
WHAT A POSITIVE EXPERIENCE A CAESAREAN CAN BE

Every birthing experience is different. Mostly, every mother finds each of their births different too (I sure did!). I have spoken to many women who found their caesarean birth really positive and some even say it was easy.

I WISH SOMEONE HAD TOLD ME ...
THAT I COULDN'T EAT AFTER A CAESAREAN
UNTIL I PASSED WIND

Imagine you have been in labour for 18+ hours and spent a good time of that pushing for dear life, only to end up with an emergency caesarean because your little poppet wouldn't budge. Now it's all over, you are starved and want to consume the biggest burger the world has ever seen. Unfortunately, you may not be allowed. When you can eat again will depend on your hospital's policy and also your individual circumstances during the surgery, but generally food, after a caesarean, works on a reward system. Classy, as giving birth is, you will be rewarded for bodily functions. Reward for no farts and no poo = nothing, other than clear liquids; reward for passing wind = light meals; reward for a bowel movement = eat pretty much anything you like. There is a reason behind this tummy torment though. Because your intestines have been relaxed during the surgery your midwife or obstetrician need to make sure they are functioning properly again before you chow down.

I WISH SOMEONE HAD TOLD ME...
TO CHEW GUM AFTER MY CAESAREAN[5,6]

OK stay with me here, I haven't lost the plot completely, this is out-there but really interesting. As mentioned before, after a caesarean, or any abdominal surgery really, the bowels can become sluggish to the point where there can be a delay for a few days of regular bowel movements (poo-poos). This can also delay healing which means longer discomfort and longer stays in the hospital. Crazy but true, chewing gum after a caesarean can help return bowel motility quicker. It basically tricks the body into thinking you are eating and so kick-starts the digestive system again. Although this requires quite extensive and regular chewing, if it means you get more comfort quicker and out of hospital sooner, it's probably worth packing a few packets of chewy in your hospital bag just in case.

I WISH SOMEONE HAD TOLD ME...
I WOULD HAVE GAS PAIN IN MY SHOULDERS
AFTER A CAESAREAN

OK, I know this probably sounds really cray-cray but there are a bunch of women that I have spoken to who will attest to this. Gas, aka fart/wind/fluff pain can happen when your bowels become lethargic after your caesarean surgery (that's why your first poo is oh so interesting to your caregivers). These feelings of cheek squeak can be felt even in your shoulders (!!!) due to actual trapped gas or thanks to a medical phenomenon called referred pain[7]. This means the pain is sent from other parts of your body, such as your uterus or tummy muscles. You probably couldn't give two hoots about that at the time because it can hurt immensely, but it usually only lasts a short while. You may be offered some medicine to help reduce the gas, or you could just whack a chewy in your gob.

IMMEDIATELY AFTER BIRTH

I WISH SOMEONE HAD TOLD ME ...
HOW TOTALLY MESSY CHILDBIRTH IS

Some things in life we should really be warned about. This is one of them... You may be aware that having a baby is messy but probably not the extent of messiness involved. After my first boy was born Hubs dared to go down "the other end" (cue scary music!). He said it looked like I had been attacked by a grizzly bear. And that's just the blood and gashes. Throw into the mix poo, pee, sweat, tears, vomit, vernix and bucket loads of amniotic fluid, and you have yourself one very normal, natural childbirth.

I WISH SOMEONE HAD TOLD ME ...
HOW AMAZING I WOULD FEEL RIGHT AFTER GIVING BIRTH

I don't know if this is specific to my births but immediately after all three of my babies "popped" out I felt unbelievable. I was ecstatic.

I was in awe of them, in awe of myself and my body, and in awe of the miracle of childbirth. It hit me every time. I felt the most amazing joy which I shared with everyone in the room because I became so chatty (probably too chatty ☺). Hormones are going crazy through your body at this point but the feeling is indescribable. So, so wonderful, just like your newborn baby. It lasts a little while but eventually you do come back down to earth. For me it was never a crash though; more just a general feeling I settled into. Good times!

I WISH SOMEONE HAD TOLD ME ...
HOW EXHAUSTED I WOULD BE AFTER GIVING BIRTH

Once the initial ecstasy settles, exhaustion can really set in. Giving birth is no mean feat. No matter how your baby comes into the world, it is exhausting for both mum and bub. If you add a long and arduous labour on top of that, perhaps with a long pushing phase, followed by a possible emergency caesarean, it is not surprising some women are absolutely shattered after giving birth. Having said that, pushing out a baby in the quickest and most straight-forward way is also very taxing. "Hit by a truck" came up often in this context when I was speaking to mums. Although bloody hard work, I felt OK after having my three (even the naughty little #1 monster) so it really varies from mum to mum. Rest assured (yes, pun intended!) no matter how exhausted you are after giving birth, you will find more energy once it's all over to shower your little one with cuddles and kisses.

I WISH SOMEONE HAD TOLD ME...
HOW WOBBLY MY LEGS WOULD FEEL

Wobbly legs are not restricted to women who have had epidurals or spinal blocks. Drug-free and/or vaginal births make your legs like jelly too. There is a reason they give you your baby in that big plastic bassinet on wheels: to steady you when you walk to the toilet or the dining room. Think of it as a new mother's walking frame! Just kidding of course, that's not what babies (or their bassinets) are for, they're to keep you awake for the next eight years. Ha ha ha!

I WISH SOMEONE HAD TOLD ME...
I WOULD SHAKE UNCONTROLLABLY

Like wobbly legs, shaking can occur whether you had an epidural, spinal block, no drugs, caesarean or vaginal birth. I had it really bad when I finally got that spinal block (as they were stitching me new again) after my first baby, but never while I was, or soon after, giving birth. Or at least not severe enough for me to notice through my state of yay-it's-finally-over elation. I felt really cold during the spinal block shaking. Some mums do too, whereas some just shake. What causes the actual shaking is still largely unknown[8]. I have heard from mums that they found the shaking to be worse when they had an epidural for a C-section, as opposed to an epidural for a vaginal birth, which I find so interesting. The shaking can get really severe in some cases and I have heard a few times now that new mums were afraid to hold their babies for fear of dropping them. Not that they could communicate this because their teeth were chattering so badly (some mums even bite their tongue or lips). Luckily the extreme shaking doesn't last too long, then you can have your well-deserved first cuddle and normal conversation again.

I WISH SOMEONE HAD TOLD ME ...
I MAY NOT GET TO HOLD MY BABY STRAIGHT AWAY

If you had a general anaesthetic (which is very rare these days) this is probably a given as you need to wake up before you can hold your bub, but sometimes there are other scenarios when your brand new baby may be handed over to medical staff instead of you. A premature birth, complications during delivery or meconium in your waters are all reasons you may have to wait for your first cuddles. Although it may cause you some anxiety that your baby is not in your arms, please know that the best people are looking after your little one and she will be getting mummy-cuddles as soon as possible.

I WISH SOMEONE HAD TOLD ME ...
TO SPECIFY WHO GETS TO HOLD MY BABY

With the exception of medical staff of course (because they are all about looking after your baby and are not in it for the cuddles), it is totally OK to put a note in your birth plan about who can hold the baby if the case arises that you can't. A friend of mine unfortunately needed a general anaesthetic with the birth of her first baby. This was, of course, not planned so she hadn't even thought about what would happen to her baby while she was in recovery. Turns out her family and in-laws had a small celebration in her room while she was waking up in recovery and her new baby was being passed around to second aunts and twice-removed cousins before she even had a chance to meet him. Even five years later she is still sad that her brother in-law's girlfriend's (who he is no longer with!) sister got to hold her boy before she did. Her fury and dismay is totally understandable, I think.

I WISH SOMEONE HAD TOLD ME...
THAT THE BABY AND PLACENTA ARE NOT THE ONLY THINGS I'D BE PUSHING OUT – HAEMORRHOIDS!

Well, when you push that hard and long it is inevitable that something else will be pushed out too. I think we have covered the poo and pee, that comes with pushing, enough for one sitting but I must mention haemorrhoids at this point, because it would be rude not to. So basically, haemorrhoids are varicose veins of the rectum, and while you may have encountered them during your pregnancy, they will probably also make an entrance (or rather exit!) during the pushing phase. A husband I spoke to about this wonderful topic told me his wife's bum looked like a minefield after she gave birth to their son. Unfortunately, they can stick around for a while after your baby is born which makes number 2s oh so frightening (stock up on stool softeners!!!) but they will go away eventually. I promise. They will. Eventually.

I WISH SOMEONE HAD TOLD ME ...
HOW INCREDIBLY HUNGRY I WOULD BE AFTER GIVING BIRTH

It's not called labour for nothin'. Giving birth is hard work. And hard work makes you very, very, very hungry. Hopefully by the time your baby has arrived any kind of nausea will have subsided and you can enjoy a delicious tray of hospital food. Yum! No seriously, hospital food will taste alright at this point. Or you can send your partner on a food run. After all three of my kids Hubs brought me prawns, sashimi, cured meats, oysters and soft cheeses. Every mum deserves a reward for a job well done. Enjoy girlfriend!

FIRST FEW HOURS AFTER BIRTH

I WISH SOMEONE HAD TOLD ME ...
THAT PERINEAL STITCHES CAN TAKE A WHILE

Oh my, the whole stitching process after a vaginal birth can drag on and on and on and on and on... well, you get the picture. With my first I was rushed to theatre to have the damage repaired so it was understandable that it all took a bit longer. But with my second, stitching (of what I was assured were only a few small grazes) took, what seemed like, forever. I have heard this from many mothers and wonder whether it is the perception that it takes a long time because you have just given birth, you're a bit out of it (in a good way!) and all you want to do is curl up with your newborn and cuddle it silly. Or that the sterility of the process: gloves, bright lights and surgery material make it so unpleasant you just can't wait to get out of there. Either way, half an hour plus with your legs spread in a doctor's or midwife's face is not uncommon, so be prepared. On the upside, if all went well and baby is OK you might be able to cuddle your newborn during the stitching process.

THAT THE FIRST ATTEMPT AT STITCHING MAY NOT BE THE LAST

Like placing an epidural, stitching of the perineum can sometimes also not go perfectly the first time around. While you are lying with your legs spread, and/or in stirrups, and your va-jay-jay is in the air for all to see, the last thing you want to hear is your caregiver contemplating re-doing the stitches because they want to do them a little tighter or not quite so tight. Say what!?!? Because we are all only human, it does happen, but a little extra time and discomfort at that point is better than a botched perineum from here on in. Think of the consequences! Your lady garden will never look the same again as it is, you don't want it to be completely disfigured and defective, do you?

THAT THE FIRST PAIN RELIEF FOR MY STITCHES WILL BE ADMINISTERED ANALLY[9]

Yes, these pain meds go up your bum! Having something shoved up your tush when you have just given birth may be the last thing you feel like; the area is sensitive, swollen and sore. However, the person stitching you new again will administer it so swiftly you won't even know it happened. And you won't feel it once it is up there.

I WISH SOMEONE HAD TOLD ME…
THAT MY CATHETER WILL STAY IN FOR A WHILE AFTER I HAVE GIVEN BIRTH

Unfortunately, following an epidural or spinal block you won't have good use of your legs for a little while, so you can't trot off to the toot whenever nature calls. The catheter will stay inserted until the anaesthetic has fully worn off and you can skip to the loo once again. This can be up to 24 hours after your anaesthetic. So enjoy the lie-in, it'll probably be your last for a while.

I WISH SOMEONE HAD TOLD ME…
TO ASK FOR A LAXATIVE AS MY FIRST POST-DELIVERY MEDICINE

So depending on how you birthed your little cherub, and how willingly they were born, each mother is likely to have varying levels of discomfort (*read:* pain) when they return to the hospital ward. The midwives will be quite obliging in offering you pain medicine for your tear/graze/incision/fractured tail bone/bruised va-jay-jay etc., and by all means take it but make sure you ask for a laxative as well. Your first bowel movement (aka fudge baby) is extremely fascinating to your midwife (especially if you had a caesarean) and they will ask you often if you have done a number 2 yet. Remember this indicates your intestines are OK post-birth. So you want to poo and you want to poo soon. There is just one problem. The utter fear that pulsates through your body at the mere thought of sending the kids to the pool. I mean think of what just happened down there and now you are meant to do what?!?! Seriously, ask for a laxative! If nothing else, it will take the edge off your justified anxiety. Oh and when the time comes, a strategically pressed wad of toilet paper on your damaged nether region will make the poo process a little more comfortable too.

I WISH SOMEONE HAD TOLD ME ...
THAT THE FIRST SHOWER AFTER GIVING BIRTH WOULD BE THE BEST SHOWER I HAVE EVER HAD IN MY LIFE

There is really not much more to add to this. You will experience it for yourself. The only disclaimer is that "down there" (or your C-section scar!) is very tender and fragile, but other than that. Best. Shower. Ever.

I WISH SOMEONE HAD TOLD ME ...
THAT MY STOMACH WOULD BE PUSHED A LOT AFTER GIVING BIRTH

Oh yes, happy birth day! The wonderful journey of childbirth continues. Now that everything that needs to be out of you is out, your stretched-to-its-limits uterus is of prime concern. Your midwife will push and prod your stomach a lot to ensure your uterus is shrinking at the desired rate, indicating everything is A-OK. Also known as a uterine fundal massage, the prodding serves other purposes too: not only will any material still inside be expelled, but your midwife can also feel any abnormalities through the skin which can be attended to before things become dire. Verdict: annoying, because of its frequency, but not really painful in itself (think of what you've just been through!).

I WISH SOMEONE HAD TOLD ME ...
THAT PEEING WOULD BE SO SCARY

What can I say? Huge trauma in the vaginal area + urine = stingy! Drink lots of water to dilute the stinginess. It doesn't last too long but some tricks you could try in the meantime are:

- Relieving yourself in the shower. While the shower is on of course, otherwise that would defeat the purpose (no, golden showers will not come to mind, you will be too sore and scared!)

- Leaning backwards so the stream of pee is re-directed away from your tender area.

• Filling a spouted drink bottle with lukewarm, very lightly salted water and squirting that like it's going out of fashion while you do your number 1s. This bottle is also a good friend after you do number 2s. You gotta keep that area clean!

I WISH SOMEONE HAD TOLD ME ...
THAT DOING POOS WOULD TERRIFY ME

If you think peeing was scary, wait until you need to do your first poo. It literally will scare the crap out of you (if only!). I found that if you get a whole wad of toilet paper and gently press it against your graze/stitches/generally sore area, the whole pooing experience is not quite as traumatic as the mind would like to think. Having said that, still ask for a gentle laxative as soon as you hit the ward. Trust me!

I WISH SOMEONE HAD TOLD ME ...
ABOUT THE EXTENT OF SWELLING AND BRUISING
DOWN THERE

Two words: DON'T LOOK!!! While it is somewhat logical – trauma trauma trauma!!! – nobody can really prepare you for what you may see if you are game with a handheld mirror. But take it from me, you *don't* want to see it. You won't be able to unsee it! Is it too nasty to call giving birth vagina battery? There is everything from cuts and grazes to bruises and swelling, varicose veins (yes, around and inside your vagina and bum), even grizzly bear-like tears if you are unlucky like me. If I talked about the "injuries" in any other context, people would feel very sorry for you, but since it's childbirth it is beautiful – which all jokes aside, it really is. But nope, I think vagina battery is pretty much spot on.

I WISH SOMEONE HAD TOLD ME ...
ABOUT FROZEN MATERNITY PADS

I *really* wish somebody had told me about these things because after my first whopper tore me to shreds, I really could have used one. Apparently some hospitals have them available. I never got one (cue: sad face), but maybe ask your midwife if your hospital does, especially if you too had a "how-you-goin'" birth like mine. You can also make them at home when you leave the hospital which might be nice (although knowledge that has come a little too late for me). From what I hear they are the bees' knees. I can only imagine the relief!

THE FIRST
FEW WEEKS
AFTER

HEALING AFTER GIVING BIRTH

I WISH SOMEONE HAD TOLD ME...
NOT TO LOOK "DOWN THERE"

I know we already covered this in the delivery section of this book, but I thought it is worthy to mention again: avoid looking at your lady garden after you have given birth. It isn't pretty. It is carnage! And not limited to your vagina. Your bum gets a pretty good workout too. Black and blue, doesn't begin to cover it. Even days or weeks after you have given birth this area will still be recovering, that includes the bruising, grazes, stitches etc. If you do look, don't say I didn't warn you.

I WISH SOMEONE HAD TOLD ME ...
THAT I WILL CONTINUE TO HAVE CONTRACTIONS AFTER MY BABY IS BORN

After pains, aka clearly-you-haven't-suffered-enough-yet pains, are very common while breastfeeding the first few days after giving birth. It is part of the body's natural process to contract your uterus. Not that knowing that will make them any less painful. They can really rock you, particularly in the first day or two of breastfeeding. Your midwife may even offer you pain relief to take the edge off. More bad news on this topic is that most women say after pains are worse with each subsequent baby. I agree. Yippee!!!

I WISH SOMEONE HAD TOLD ME ...
NOT TO WEIGH MYSELF AFTER GIVING BIRTH

OK, I'll tell you: do not weigh yourself after giving birth. You will be bitterly disappointed...

I WISH SOMEONE HAD TOLD ME ...
THAT MY BELLY WOULD NOT SHRINK INSTANTLY AFTER MY BABY IS BORN

I have two words for you: Kate Middleton. Remember when she emerged from the hospital all coiffed after the birth of Princess

Charlotte, and she looked seven months pregnant? Yeah, if Princess Catherine can't get rid of her baby belly instantly, then there is no hope for any of us. I know it looks like there is another baby hiding in there but alas it is just the norm. Remember as far as weight and your figure is concerned: nine months on, nine months off. Oh and make a mental note to pack maternity clothes for your hospital stay and your trip home. Or at least clothes you wore at seven or eight months pregnant, because your pre-baby clothes are unlikely to fit around your tum for the first little while post-baby.

I WISH SOMEONE HAD TOLD ME ...
ABOUT ALL THE LOCHIA

The what??? The blood! The blood! The post-baby blood!!! Lochia is as glamorous as it sounds, I'm afraid. It's the expulsion of the lining of your massive uterus which you no longer need. This happens whether you had a vaginal or caesarean delivery. Good-o! Lochia will start vacating your va-jay-jay a few hours after you have given birth for about six weeks. Hooray! It is like having a period with a vengeance. The consistency is the same as when Flo visits but there is oh so much and it can be filled with clots! You will be surprised that pads come in *that* size, that you can fill them and that you can bleed so long and intensely without repercussions. You may be shocked (or completely freaked out) at the size of the clots. If one plops in the toilet while you're on there you may wonder if you have just delivered another baby, or your intestines fell out of your clacker. Yes, they can be that big! When your nurse checks on you she may peek in your pants to see how full your pad is. It's really quite disgusting (the blood, not the nurse), but oh so wonderful at the same time. Your body carried a baby! You are now a fully-fledged mum (with maternity pads the size of surfboards that need to be changed regularly for weeks. Oh the glamour)! All I can say is, make sure you stock up on those massive maternity pads and old granny undies (especially when you are still in hospital). And try not to get too attached to said gigantic underwear as chances are you will need to chuck them when you're done ☺.

I WISH SOMEONE HAD TOLD ME ...
HOW CONSTIPATED I WOULD BE

Yes, it's those hormones again (the troublesome things that they are!). But it could also be due to the pain medication you had during labour (many of those make you constipated), or just labour itself (the digestive system slows down dramatically during labour), amongst other things. Have I mentioned stool softeners, aka laxatives? I think only about 10 times. Take them. Religiously. From day one. You do not want to get to the loo and realise that, after everything your poor nether regions have been through, your first poo is a very solid one. There is a rumour that your first bowel movement actually won't hurt. That's a lie! If you're anything like me and sustained quite the trauma while giving birth, you won't want to find out. Just take your stool softener, even if just for peace of mind, otherwise you may be punching a hole in the wall while you're backing the big brown bus out of the garage.

I WISH SOMEONE HAD TOLD ME ...
THAT DOING A NUMBER 2 WILL SCARE ME SO MUCH

Nicely moving into this from my lovely constipation story… Poos are scary, OK!?! Right after you've had a baby, a couple of days later, even a few weeks later. All the stuff that has gone on down there and the things that have come out down there (hae-mate-roids) can make sending the kids to the pool a frightening concept. Especially when you are rather constipated. Rest assured you will not rip yourself a new hole, nor will your insides come out your bum or elsewhere. Your stitches will remain intact and so will you. There is no need to take someone to the toilet with you, you will survive. Stay strong, grab the stool softener and proceed. Remember that strategically placed toilet paper can help and if you end up letting out a little yelp or a big cry, like me, know that this won't last forever and you too will look back on it one day. Although it may take a while until you can laugh about it.

I WISH SOMEONE HAD TOLD ME ...
THAT HAEMORRHOIDS MAY STICK AROUND
AFTER GIVING BIRTH

I know, way too much information! But you're reading this book, so I am guessing you really do want to know. Haemorrhoids don't always disappear after you have your baby. And by that I mean they can stick around or stick out (if you prefer) for a *while* (like months!!!) after you have given birth. As they're varicose, i.e. swollen, veins of the anus (super, thanks for sharing!), they will disappear when the swelling subsides. Just in case you weren't grossed out enough, I had them post all three of my kidlets. They made doing number 2s so painful (the haemorrhoids that is, not the kids), even weeks after I had given birth. I remember there were a couple of times I even cried during a bowel movement, and yes, I was already on the laxatives. Some say push them back in, some say let them hang out, either way try and minimise the time they call your bum their home by looking after yourself (and them).

I WISH SOMEONE HAD TOLD ME ...
HOW LONG I WOULD BE IN PAIN FOR AFTER GIVING BIRTH

It may seem a little more self-explanatory with caesarean births because it's major surgery, and you expect some healing of the incision. However, if you have a vaginal birth, you will soon understand that that needs to heal too. Of course it depends on the type of birth you had as to the extent of healing required. After my first baby I couldn't sit down properly for quite a while. The couch or anything soft was fine but when Hubs kindly took me out to lunch a few days after getting home from hospital, the bench seats at the trendy Café were too much for me to bear. Luckily, the woman running the place seemed to have a couple of kids under her belt because when she saw us coming with this tiny munchkin, and saw me struggle to sit, she pulled a massive cushion out of her hat (a perfect example of The Secret Mothers' club mentioned later). Walking was pretty tricky for a while too.

I have even spoken to women who said they had trouble lying down after having their bub. Ouch! It won't necessarily always happen to that extent (I was much better after I had my other two) but probably best not to book in a 10km fun run in the first few weeks after your due date, just in case.

I WISH SOMEONE HAD TOLD ME...
THAT AN EPIDURAL COULD GIVE ME SUCH A HEADACHE

A post-dural puncture headache is rare, but it happened to a friend of mine so I thought it is definitely worth a mention. Headaches after giving birth are common. A dural headache is different because it is so severe (apparently it's really more like a migraine than a headache), and the pain is worse when standing or sitting, compared to lying down. It is due to a small puncture in the dura (the outermost layer of the spinal cord) after you receive an epidural or spinal block. However, you probably won't feel the pain in your head until after you have had your baby. There are things that can help, one of which is lots of caffeine, which if you are breastfeeding can make things very interesting. #BouncingBaby

Note: this is only funny once the dural puncture has mended and you are pain free!

I WISH SOMEONE HAD TOLD ME ...
HOW HOT AND SWEATY I WOULD BE

I know what you're thinking, but no this is not the bit where we talk about having sex again post-baby. Nor is it the sexy hot, as in "you're hawt, girlfriend!". Nah-huh, it is the gross, sweaty, just-ran-for-a-bus-on-a-35-degree-day perspiration type of hot. Postnatal sweating will mainly happen at night (maybe put your favourite pillow to the side for a while) and should only last a few weeks. It can also be followed by chills because sweating alone isn't uncomfortable enough (jokes!). Like most things postnatal, these hot flashes are driven by hormones (surprise, surprise!) and do serve a purpose. Although disgusting, the sweating rids your body of excess fluid retained during pregnancy. The glamour continues!

I WISH SOMEONE HAD TOLD ME ...
I WOULD PEE MORE THAN USUAL

You've just been pregnant for 40-odd weeks, so I don't know what peeing more than usual actually means. When you're pregnant you're a peeing machine, right? At least in the beginning and end of it all. Anyway, I digress. You will go for number 1s more than you are used to after having your baby because this is another way for the body to get rid of excess fluid. In this instance via the kidneys i.e. more pee-pees. So, really for the first little while you'll just be peeing and sweating and feeding and peeing and sweating and feeding... ☺ Don't drink less water though, your body still needs plenty of fluid, especially if you're breastfeeding.

I WISH SOMEONE HAD TOLD ME...
HOW UNGLAMOROUS I WOULD FEEL

OK, unglamorous is an understatement. Forget the Hollywood movies or images in magazines. In the days and months after giving birth you will have times when you feel totally gross. You will probably still be carrying extra weight, your hair will be falling out, you're sweating like a rhino (do rhinos even sweat?), your skin may still be blotchy, you have haemorrhoids and varicose veins, milk soaked patches on your shirt and are bleeding for your country. If you can make that look glamorous my hat goes off to you. If you can't, you are in very good company. But it is okay, this phase passes too and you will feel sexy again. One day.

I WISH SOMEONE HAD TOLD ME...
HOW SEXY I WOULD FEEL

We are all such different creatures, aren't we? What is totally unglamorous for some is super sexy for another. Some women find that the feeling they get, knowing what their body has achieved, far outweighs the yuck feeling of extra baby weight. For other women the extra kilos and increase in cup size are welcomed with open arms. Hormones may also still be at play here. Some women are so turned on by these changes that they cannot wait to jump in the sack with their partner once they have been given the green light by their doctor. Lucky them, I say, because for me it was much, much more unglamorous than that. Ask Hubs, he'll tell you!

I WISH SOMEONE HAD TOLD ME ...
HOW WEAK MY PELVIC FLOOR WOULD BE

Farts on the loose!!! Now that I have your attention, let's revisit this very important topic. Please do your pelvic floor exercises when you are pregnant (or preferably also before you're pregnant). You will thank me later. After birth, your pelvic floor is stretched and weakened. It is responsible for keeping your bladder and bowel under control. Yes, that means: weak pelvic floor = less control of pees and poos making an unplanned escape. And most of all farts (I wasn't kidding with my first sentence). After you've given birth, farts can just breakout without warning. The whole area down there is weaker and holding a fluff in can be *really* hard. As my midwife always said to me: pelvic floor exercises, pelvic floor exercises, pelvic floor exercises. DO THEM NOW!

I WISH SOMEONE HAD TOLD ME ...
I WOULD BE AFRAID TO SNEEZE

Or cough, lift anything, exercise etc.... Your pelvic floor has been through the wringer (no pun intended there). The thought of a simple sneeze can be terrifying. Is my pelvic floor strong enough to not let anything escape? Pelvic floor problems after birth are very, very common but generally if you keep doing your exercises, you should be able to eliminate any issues or possibly reduce the severity. As I said: DO THEM NOW! However, if your pelvic floor is very weak and the exercises don't seem to make a difference, there are lots of professionals out there that can help.

I WISH SOMEONE HAD TOLD ME ...
ABOUT STOMACH MUSCLE SEPARATION

It's over!!!! Well sort of, our stomach muscles have just separated, not broken up. Ha ha! It's really called diastasis recti and basically means that as your belly gets bigger your stomach muscles move to either side because your uterus is putting more pressure on them. Although it is very common, it doesn't happen to everyone. The good news: your belly has more room to grow without the restriction of your six-pack. The bad news: amongst other things, it can lead to back pain and pelvic instability, i.e. you could pee yourself a little when you next have a big belly laugh. Get your caregiver to check your separation at your six-week post-birth appointment. While you might be pleasantly surprised to find you have none or very little, it's best to get onto it ASAP if there is still some larger separation, just to prevent any further and ongoing problems.

RECOVERY SPECIFIC TO CAESAREAN DELIVERIES

I WISH SOMEONE HAD TOLD ME …
I WILL BOND WITH MY BABY AFTER HAVING A CAESAREAN

There have been some studies done on bonding, comparing mothers who had their baby via caesarean versus a vaginal delivery. Small studies suggest that women who have C-sections take longer to bond with their baby as less hormones are released when one has a caesarean delivery. Even the researchers in this particular study[10] say the study number is small (it consisted of 12 mums) and while the results are significant, the numbers are not overwhelming. They also say that a few months later there was basically no difference seen in "bonding" hormones between the two groups. Now, I have spoken to a lot of women (more than 12!) who have had caesarean births, that had no problem bonding with their baby immediately. Similarly, I have spoken to some women who had vaginal births that did not bond with their baby straight away. I am not poo-pooing the study by any means (I love science!), it is definitely worth knowing, but we are all individuals and I think we should keep that in mind too.

I WISH SOMEONE HAD TOLD ME ...
I WOULD NOT BE ABLE TO DO ANYTHING FOR SO LONG AFTER HAVING A CAESAREAN

Your doctor will probably recommend you don't do anything that involves lifting, stretching or bending for about six weeks after you have a C-section. That includes driving, unfortunately. It is a major operation after all, and you can do some serious damage if you don't listen to this one. I know many fit, young, new mums who thought they could get back on their feet much sooner than the recommended time only to find an infection at their incision site. Incision is incision, no matter what your age or fitness level. Please be wise, get some help in the house and enjoy the down time. Once your baby is a toddler you will be wishing you could sit still for just one minute again.

I WISH SOMEONE HAD TOLD ME ...
HOW MUCH IT HURTS TO REMOVE THE DRESSING FROM MY CAESAREAN SCAR

Is it like removing a Band-Aid? On a much larger, and much stickier, scale I have heard it sort of is. But let's not forget it is on an area that has just undergone major surgery. #Ouch! I have heard swabbing the area with a nice oil, like olive, baby or coconut oil, can reduce some of the pain. Sticky stuff hates oil, you see. But other than that I have not heard of any other tips except: don't forcibly remove it and good luck!

I WISH SOMEONE HAD TOLD ME ...
MY CAESAREAN SCAR WOULD BE SO PAINFUL

Recovery after a C-section can take some time. After all, it is an operation so pain at the incision site soon after you have your baby is a given. However, some women I have spoken to told me that they experienced pain for some time after they had their baby. This can be isolated to where your incision is or referred pain to other areas. Some women said that they have a feeling of being pulled forward which can cause backache. Please mention it to your caregiver, even if it has been some time since your birth, but know that this can be part of a normal recovery.

I WISH SOMEONE HAD TOLD ME ...
MY CAESAREAN SCAR CAN AFFECT MY DIGESTION

It is rare but the tightening caused by the scar tissue of your C-section can pull into the abdominal cavity which can affect your internal organs. This can lead to an upset tummy or more unpleasant things like irritable bowel syndrome or constipation[11]. Usually if your scar is treated to be more flexible this can be reversed. There are some amazing professionals out there that can help you with this.

I WISH SOMEONE HAD TOLD ME …
MY CAESAREAN SCAR COULD BECOME INFECTED

A friend of mine was rushed back to hospital a few days after coming home with her second baby because her scar got so infected. She had to stay in hospital even longer and they had to basically re-stitch some of the scar after cleaning it up. She is conscientious, so I'm certain she would have looked after it, but sometimes things like this are unavoidable. Please try and be vigilant!

I WISH SOMEONE HAD TOLD ME …
SCARY THINGS CAN HAPPEN TO MY CAESAREAN SCAR

Like spontaneous haematomas! Which is bleeding under the incision site due to a burst blood vessel, leaving very sore bruise-like spot. Or your scar can become slightly raised or red in colour. After all your C-section scar is like any other scar from an operation, so it can turn all sorts of shades and textures. Please keep an eye on it, you don't want to get an infection.

I WISH SOMEONE HAD TOLD ME ...
MY CAESAREAN SCAR WOULD BE NUMB AND/OR ITCHY FOR A LONG TIME

Healing from a major operation always takes some time and a caesarean is no exception. The scar tissue can be numb and/or itchy while it is healing and sometimes even for a long time after. Annoying yes, but not life-threatening and not painful, so one of the lesser evils of childbirth.

I WISH SOMEONE HAD TOLD ME ...
THAT IT WOULD TAKE THAT LONG TO RECOVER FROM A CAESAREAN

I know we covered this before but some women do find that the recovery after a C-section can take a long time, so I thought I should add a small paragraph here too. It is perfectly normal to not bounce back immediately, or in the first few days. Remember it is major surgery and there are lots of abdominal layers that are cut through to get to your baby. You will only feel like you have been hit by a truck for a while, it won't last forever. I know I haven't had a caesarean, but I do believe all the mums out there who have had caesareans and told me it's true. Be kind to yourself.

BOOBS, MILK AND BREASTFEEDING

I WISH SOMEONE HAD TOLD ME ...
HOW WEEPY I WOULD GET WHEN MY MILK IS COMING IN

O.M.G!!!! The baby blues... that was a tough time for me, and is for many, many mums. They kick in around three days after you've had your baby, when your hormones are starting to change yet again, and your massive boobs are getting bigger and starting to produce breastmilk (you will probably re-evaluate the word massive after you see how big your boobs will be when said milk is actually "in"). I was really quite weepy, especially with my first, and anything from cute ducklings in a tissue advert to the sheer sight of my post-baby thighs made me cry. Some women get weepier than others but for me the stand out difference was I never actually felt depressed, as such. The baby blues usually only last a few days (until your massive boobs have become ginormous!) so if you feel blue for a period longer than that, it's probably best to speak to your GP, health care nurse or midwife. I write about this very important topic a bit more later, but if you are feeling unusually blue, especially after the baby blues *should* have passed, please seek help. Postpartum depression (PPD) is quite common (about 1 in 7 women experience it) and it is well researched[12]. There is a lot of help out there. Please speak up. There is nothing wrong with you. Nobody will judge you. You are not a bad mother. You are just adjusting to this massive thing your body has achieved: you've given life, what a big change. Please be kind to yourself.

Just on a side note, men can suffer from PPD too[12], so make sure you keep an eye on your significant other.

I WISH SOMEONE HAD TOLD ME …
THAT MY MILK COMING IN COULD BE SO PAINFUL

Have a look in the mirror around day three or four; these are your milk jugs! Your baby is new and your boobs don't know how much milk to make yet, so they hit you with the mother lode. Your boobs will feel very sore, rock hard and even hot. You will hear the word engorged *a lot*. It could be uncomfortable for you to sleep on your side or even sit up. Some women say it is worse than labour (they must have had better labours than me). The best thing you can do is keep breastfeeding (although cabbage leaves and iced nappies help too), even though it may seem awkward and painful. Luckily engorgement only lasts about a week or so. Your baby breastfeeding signals to your boobs how much milk bub needs, and after a while your breasts will make just the right amount i.e. reduced engorgement, pain and size. Yippee!!! On the downside (sort of!), this is also the time when you and your baby are learning to breastfeed, so a few people, like your midwife or lactation consultant, will handle your engorged knockers frequently. See even here, engorged was said *a lot*. Be prepared!

I WISH SOMEONE HAD TOLD ME ...
THAT MILK CAN TAKE A WHILE TO COME IN

Usually milk "comes in" within 72 hours of giving birth, but because we humans are complex creatures this can sometimes be delayed. Some mothers told me it took up to seven days for their milk to come in. This shouldn't indicate anything but it may make you feel stressed. The milk you produce, the quality and the volume, won't be affected because it is late. The only thing that will affect your ability to breastfeed is stress. Stress can reduce your milk's flow. However, the hormone oxytocin which is released during breastfeeding can have a calming effect. So if your milk is late, don't stress, keep feeding colostrum (and getting those doses of oxytocin to make you feel Zen) and know your milk is on its way.

I WISH SOMEONE HAD TOLD ME ...
THAT WHEN MY MILK COMES IN MY BOOBS WOULD GET THAT BIG

Milk, milk and more milk. I am not sure I have described the sheer size of your milk jugs well enough, so let me be blunt: you are now preparing to become a cow in more ways than one. Think udders... I can't think of a word bigger than ginormous but your boobs will reach that level of big-ness. Lovely if you were an A-cup pre-baby, not so great when you had melons to begin with.

I WISH SOMEONE HAD TOLD ME ...
THAT MY BOOBS WOULD BE SQUEEZED A LOT

Don't get me wrong I am very grateful for the lactation help I got at the hospital with all three of my babies. But be prepared that many hands will make their way to your bosoms when you and your baby are learning to breastfeed. Often. Like each feed (which is every two hours or so!). Your already sensitive (and massive!) boobs are probably going to be prodded, squeezed or squashed to encourage let-down, aid your milk production or assist with getting the right attachment. In all honestly, they will probably get prodded, squeezed *and* squashed. It is helpful but it can hurt (a lot!) especially when your milk is coming in.

I WISH SOMEONE HAD TOLD ME ...
THAT BREASTFEEDING IS HARD

OMG breastfeeding can be so hard in the beginning. Going back to my trusty resource Hollywood, where women just put their baby towards the breast and hey presto… Oh no, no, no, no, it is so not like that. Especially with your first child as you are both in unfamiliar territory. You don't know anything and your baby is just going by instinct. It is really, really hard but so worth the cracked and bleeding nipples in the beginning to get it right. Make sure you get good advice in the hospital or see a lactation consultant if you are struggling. If you can get off to a good start it can save you so much blood, sweat and tears (literally all three), and mastitis, if you're really unlucky. Also remember that it can take a while as your baby is learning too. My second son couldn't create a vacuum (on boob or bottle) until he was 12 weeks old. It was a tough time because it was so hard to feed him but I am happy I persevered as I find breastfeeding (when it works) one of the most amazing things in the world. I know there are women out there that disagree, and I totally appreciate that but if you want to breastfeed be ready for some hard yards and perseverance.

I WISH SOMEONE HAD TOLD ME ...
TO BE CAREFUL WHEN PUMPING TO DRAW OUT THE NIPPLES

Some women have inverted or flat nipples, and this can make breastfeeding difficult. Sometimes it is recommended that you use your breast pump to draw the nipples out. I have heard from a few women now that this advice should come with a label. WARNING: don't pump too much. Increased pumping → increased milk production → enough milk to feed the street and of course super massive boobs i.e. engorgement (since we haven't heard the word nearly enough in this section already ☺).

I WISH SOMEONE HAD TOLD ME ...
I WOULD EASILY BREASTFEED AFTER HAVING A CAESAREAN

A friend of mine had a scheduled caesarean recently. Throughout her pregnancy "well-wishers" and "kind strangers" told her that she would have trouble breastfeeding after her caesarean. Great tip, thanks folks! It stressed her out a lot (as you can imagine) but once her baby was here she fed like a champ, right from the beginning. For some reason people thought (and some well-wishers still do) that a C-section slows your milk coming in. Not true! Milk starts being produced when the placenta is delivered; which happens no matter how you birth your baby. Provided your baby gets the paediatrician's OK and you are up for it, you may even start feeding in the operating room while they are stitching you up. Which of course gets you bonding, so it's a win–win. Having said that, if you have a caesarean and choose not to breastfeed, it doesn't mean you won't bond with your baby instantly. Bonding skin-on-skin contact is blissful, nurturing and such a wonderful way to start your life together.

I WISH SOMEONE HAD TOLD ME ...
THAT LET-DOWN CAN BE UNCOMFORTABLE

Usually the feeling of your let-down reflex is described as pins and needles, but in the beginning it can be a little more unpleasant, like a sharpish pain. It really does get better as time goes on. While severe pain can indicate that you may have a fast let-down, it can also signal that there is something wrong like mastitis or a thrush infection. Not everyone finds the let-down uncomfortable though. I did, but I found one very deep breath was all it took to get through it in the beginning.

I WISH SOMEONE HAD TOLD ME ...
I MAY HAVE MORE BREAST TISSUE IN MY ARM PIT

Apparently it is quite common to have breast tissue all the way up into your armpit. It is something that happens during the developmental stage when *we* are still embryos. This accessory breast tissue, as it's called, may or may not produce milk and can sometimes even resemble another whole breast, including areola and nipple! For some women it is obvious even before they start breastfeeding (I met a woman who said hers was the size of a baseball), whereas other women won't know they have it until they start leaking milk from a pore in the arm pit. Not surprisingly, like your boobs, the area can be quite tender when your milk comes in and in the early breastfeeding days. Our bodies just never seize to amaze, do they?

I WISH SOMEONE HAD TOLD ME ...
THAT ANY BABY CAN MAKE MY MILK FLOW

You've just fed your baby and decided to switch on the TV while you cuddle your little one who has fallen asleep in your arms. Such a precious time! Until you channel surf to a baby crying. Suddenly your shirt is drenched... again!

In the early weeks the rise of the hormone oxytocin, brought on by the TV baby, can trigger your let-down reflex. This phenomenon does not occur to all new mothers and is not limited to babies on TV. Oxytocin may be triggered by merely looking at your baby, sitting in your usual feeding chair, smelling your baby or even thinking of your baby. It does settle over time as your let-down reflex attunes to your new bub[13] but in the meantime wear breast pads everywhere! You never know when you will see a cute baby that reminds you of your child.... #squirt

I WISH SOMEONE HAD TOLD ME ...
ABOUT BREASTMILK OVERSUPPLY AND FAST LET-DOWNS

I never had this problem but I can imagine it would be terrible hearing (and seeing) your baby gag on your milk because there is too much or it's coming too fast. You are just trying to feed him!!! Or imagine squirting about the place for no reason other than your baby cries or you walk past a picture of him. I have heard women talk about having so much supply and such a fast let-down that they squirt their baby in the face before they can get a proper latch. That does sound pretty bad, I must say. I have a friend who could only feed lying on her side, as her baby would point-blank refuse the breast otherwise – her milk supply was too fast for him. It is impossible to tell who will have lots of milk. Big boobs don't necessarily mean lots of milk. You also can't predict your let-down reflex. Oversupply and/or a fast let-down can be tricky in the early days, but everything should settle once you have established a solid feeding routine and your boobs know how much milk to make. If not, a lactation consultant can definitely help.

I WISH SOMEONE HAD TOLD ME ...
ABOUT BREASTMILK UNDERSUPPLY AND SLOW LET-DOWNS

I know a little more about this (and my boobs are not small! They are somewhat deflated now but that's a different topic). Undersupply can be disheartening. It can make you feel low (excuse the pun) because you may feel you can't nourish your baby properly. With all three of mine I ended up pumping after each feed to get my supply up. I also drank all the teas and made lactation biscuits like they were the last food on earth. It did help but it was a lot of work. Work I was willing to put in because I loved breastfeeding. However, the stress of low supply can also impact your let-down reflex. Or sometimes the let-down is just slow. You just never know what you're gonna get when it comes to your boobs and milk. There are plenty of people out there that can help you and many who have been through it before you, if you need some support. However, if it's too hard or making you depressed, don't let anyone deter you from topping-up with, or switching to, formula. Happy mummy = happy baby, no matter how they are fed. But yes, undersupply sucks big time (certainly no pun intended there).

I WISH SOMEONE HAD TOLD ME …
HOW HUNGRY I WOULD GET WHILE BREASTFEEDING

Mmmm foooood!!! Any food!!! All food!!! You are probably feeding anywhere between every two to four hours, so milk is being produced around the clock. Your metabolism is in overdrive to make milk, so naturally you feel very hungry. The beauty about this hunger is that once you get what you crave it is especially delicious. Make sure you eat a well-balanced diet though because after all, what you eat your baby eats. *But* because you are burning so many calories producing milk, you do have an extra treat up your sleeve which should not go straight to your hips ☺. Enjoy!

I WISH SOMEONE HAD TOLD ME …
HOW THIRSTY I WOULD GET WHILE BREASTFEEDING

Oh yes, make sure you have a big glass of water with you as you begin your nursing session. When your baby latches on it will probably make you extremely thirsty. The production of milk requires the extra calories (your increased hunger) and the increase in fluid (your super thirst). So, drink drink drink – I'd love to say bubbly champagne, but better make it a long, tall glass of bubbly… water.

I WISH SOMEONE HAD TOLD ME ...
THAT SOME MEDICATIONS CAN DECREASE YOUR MILK SUPPLY

The mini-pill (a progesterone only contraceptive pill) is safe to use while breastfeeding and is thought to be less likely to have an effect on milk supply. However, many mums told me that the mini-pill drastically reduced their breastmilk output. Of course, this may not happen to everyone but just something to think about when considering contraception, once you're game to attempt the horizontal tango again. Further breastmilk demons include other hormone containing meds and large amounts of alcohol and cigarettes. Things that contain pseudoephedrine like antihistamines are also breastmilk depleting. Probably not an issue for most reading this but it is something that women told me they wish they had known about, so just letting you know.

I WISH SOMEONE HAD TOLD ME ...
THAT SOME MEDICATIONS CAN INCREASE YOUR MILK SUPPLY

On the flip side, if you are struggling to get up or keep up your supply, there are things that can help boost it. From foods such as oats and brewer's yeast (yuck!!! But it works!) to supplements like fenugreek and nursing teas. Boosting your supply could be as simple as baking a batch of lactation cookies for some, while others may need a little more help. If you can't manage to boost your supply naturally there is something your GP can prescribe for you. It is an anti-nausea and vomiting drug that can have the wonderful (if you are breastfeeding!) side-effect of stimulating milk-production. It worked great for me along with all the pumping, teas, herbs and cookies, who on their own just weren't powerful enough, and I breastfed my three happily for a long time. Remember it's a last resort though, so try all the natural methods first.

I WISH SOMEONE HAD TOLD ME …
I COULD GET PREGNANT WHILE BREASTFEEDING

This is probably the most common "I wish someone had told me…" I have heard. So let me say this very clearly: BREASTFEEDING IS NOT A CONTRACEPTIVE, LADIES!!!! You *can* get pregnant while breastfeeding. If you are breastfeeding you are less fertile, not infertile! Your first post-baby egg is released before you get your first period, so you won't even know you've ovulated until your period comes. If you don't want another baby, having unprotected sex while breastfeeding is a bit like Baby-Russian roulette, you never know when your first egg will jump from the starting line. So don't be silly, put a condom on his willy (it will save you a lot of problems if you're not ready to have another baby).

I WISH SOMEONE HAD TOLD ME …
THAT BREASTFEEDING WITH MASTITIS WOULD HURT SO MUCH

Oh mastitis, you mother of a ★&^%★!!! If you haven't met this breastfeeding-mother's nemesis yet, be very thankful. Mastitis is basically a blocked milk duct that hasn't cleared properly during feeding, and the nearby breast tissue has now become inflamed. Yay!!! Its awful symptoms include a sore, red area on the boob and flu-like symptoms (which can be really intense if your mastitis is bad). Unfortunately, one of the best treatments is to keep the breast empty i.e. drain your boob, i.e. breastfeed a lot! It hurts like crazy but it does work. Just be prepared for a little more pain.

BOTTLE-FEEDING

I WISH SOMEONE HAD TOLD ME...
IT'S OK TO BOTTLE-FEED MY CHILD

I intentionally gave bottle-feeding its own heading because there is nothing wrong with bottle-feeding. Don't let people shame you if you want, choose or have to bottle-feed. At the end of the day your baby needs to be nourished and if breastfeeding doesn't work for you or you have other reasons why you can't or don't want to breastfeed, then formula is fine. There are many healthy and successful people in the world that were formula-fed from day one. Don't let anyone make you feel bad because you bottle-feed. People will shoot you dirty looks regardless of whether you stick a bottle in your baby's mouth or pull out your boob to breastfeed. In this regard you can't win – C'est la vie!

EMOTIONS

I WISH SOMEONE HAD TOLD ME ...
ABOUT THE SEVERITY OF THE BABY BLUES

Chances are you felt elated when you finally held Baby in your arms for the first time; it is such an exhilarating time. But about three days later the majority of women experience these wretched baby blues. Described as a general weepiness and irritability, it's the time when your hormones change yet again, your milk is coming in and you may wonder how on earth you can possibly look after something so little and fragile 24/7. The smallest things can set your tears rolling. One mum told me she cried out of gratitude to the staff member who brought the "yummy" hospital dinner to her bedside. These blues can be quite severe, but should pass after a few days. If you feel down for longer please, please, please talk to your doctor.

I WISH SOMEONE HAD TOLD ME ...
THAT THE CAR RIDE HOME WILL BE FILLED WITH SO MANY EMOTIONS

This part may get lost in all the antenatal and postnatal info, but the time when you take your baby home is a very special, yet scary, time. Your emotions may be all over the place – excited because you are finally taking your baby home, then scared because how on earth will you take care of a baby (what was the hospital thinking letting you take him home?), then a little apprehensive (is he okay there in such a big capsule?), then proud because you did it! Enjoy the moment whichever way it is for you, your life as a mum has well and truly begun.

I WISH SOMEONE HAD TOLD ME ...
THAT ONCE YOU HAVE A BABY YOU BECOME AN INSTANT MEMBER OF THE SECRET MOTHERS CLUB

Fight Club eat your heart out! The knowing little looks and approving nods you get from other mums when you carry, or wheel, your newborn around are amazing. You are now part of an elite group. These women know what you have been through. I remember when I had just had my first son, I was lost in a new world. I aimlessly wandered around the supermarket because I had forgotten what I came for, and was close to tears because of the "help" being hurled at me about what my baby wanted and needed. Were these advice-givers even mothers? Then I walked past two elderly women. They stopped their conversation to look at me. They smiled. They never looked at my son just at me, and they nodded. Their nods gave me such strength and reassurance I will remember this moment for as long as I live. From then on I noticed this wasn't an exception. I was part of The Secret Mothers Club and unlike Fight Club it's OK to talk about it.

I WISH SOMEONE HAD TOLD ME...
PPD IS NOT JUST DEPRESSION

Postpartum depression (PPD) is such a serious and vast topic. I won't go into it too much in this book. But because it is so important I just want to outline the following essential things... PPD can be lots of things, not just depression. I actually didn't know this, so when Hubs asked me, soon after Baby #3 was born, if I thought maybe I had PPD I dismissed it immediately; I wasn't depressed, I was stressed! It wasn't until Baby #3 was about 15 months old and I was writing this chapter of the book and extensively researching PPD that I thought maybe I had had it. Was my nervous-breakdown-due-to-severe-sleep-deprivation in fact PPD? Or specifically PPA (postpartum anxiety) in my case? I guess I will never know.

PPD and PPA can manifest as a range of feelings including[14]: low self-esteem and lack of confidence, feelings of inadequacy and guilt, negative thoughts, feelings of life being meaningless, feeling unable to cope, tearfulness and irritability, difficulty sleeping or changes in sleeping patterns (aside from baby's influence), anxiety, panic attacks or heart palpitations, loss of appetite and difficulty concentrating or remembering things.

Yes, having three kids in three-and-a-half years was a stressful event in itself, but in hindsight I certainly could identify with a lot of those feelings.

Please, please, please say something if you are not feeling OK after having your baby. Admission of such feelings is not a sign of weakness, it shows you are strong. Empower yourself by putting your hand up. You are not alone!

I WISH SOMEONE HAD TOLD ME ...
YOU CAN GET PPD AND/OR PPA WITH SUBSEQUENT KIDS WHEN YOU NEVER HAD IT BEFORE

A good friend and I had our three kids around similar times. Our first are only a couple of weeks apart in age, and our third about four weeks (but that is only because hers came two weeks early and mine was an agonising nine days late). Our third, both girls, were very similar in temperament and sleeping routines i.e. *not* sleeping at all. We spoke (*read*: complained, whinged, cried, laughed) a lot about them and compared notes. A few months in we both admitted we were really struggling. We both fought with it for a long time and sadly learned the hard way that if you avoided PPD or PPA (or your version of a nervous-breakdown-due-to-severe-sleep-deprivation) with your older child, it doesn't mean it won't hit you with your second, third, fourth or tenth. Please take care of yourself and stay on the lookout for signs. It's OK to be not OK. As I said before please speak up if you don't feel OK. This stuff can manifest in all sorts of different ways and it can pull the rug out from under you. But there are people out there that can help you; please seek them out.

PS. This does not mean you need to take medication. Sometimes a good chat with a professional can work wonders.

I WISH SOMEONE HAD TOLD ME...
I WILL GET THROUGH THE TOUGH TIMES

If you believe nothing else in this book, please believe this… one way or another you will get through the tough times, if you ask for help. Reaching out to a partner, a family member, a friend or a doctor can help so much. If you see a doctor that does not necessarily mean you have to take medication. If the thought of that makes you even more anxious or depressed, a healthy lifestyle, mindfulness, meditation, exercise and therapy can sometimes be enough to get you through. It was for me. I don't want to sound rude and judgemental, I just want to share my story… I was almost hospitalised. The psychiatrist I saw wanted to put me on anti-psychotic drugs, not just antidepressants. I was curled up in a blanket (in December! For all our foreign friends, that is summer in Australia) in a ball on my couch for weeks, only rising when my poor children were desperate for something. I had to beg my mum to stay with us because I was incapable of living (strangely though, I still managed to care for my kids). I didn't sleep more than 20 minutes at a time for months! I was petrified of everything, especially being alone with my kids (who ironically I still loved dearly). I am not judging people who choose medication, everyone is on their own journey and everyone must do what is right for them. However, I just wanted to mention that there are other options too, and they work – I am proof. These all also work very well in conjunction with medication. Just letting you know ☺.

When I was struggling, I used my science knowledge and evidence-based techniques to teach myself to thrive again. Out of this, I created my courses which, at the time of writing, have helped hundreds of mums and mums to-be thrive again. To learn more please see www.DrJen.com.au

I WISH SOMEONE HAD TOLD ME...
THAT NO MOTHER HAS IT ALL TOGETHER

It's true, we are all winging it! Please do not for one second think that other mums have it together and you don't. It doesn't matter how much of a front they put up (in fact the ones with the most perfect front are the ones that are usually struggling the most), being a mother (especially to a newborn) is tough. And honestly it doesn't matter whether it's your first, second, third or eighth child. It's OK to show vulnerability, because the truth is no mother of young kids has it all together. EVER! There, I said it.

I WISH SOMEONE HAD TOLD ME...
MY EMOTIONS WOULD CHANGE

A lot of things change when you have a baby (is that the understatement of the century?). And one of the major things for me, and many other mums, are emotions. I don't just mean the effect hormones had on me after I had my babies, I mean long-term emotions. As one of my friends put it: I *feel* more. And it happens to a lot of women. I suppose some feelings can be considered negative, such as getting teary because you saw a sad story on TV (especially anything to do with babies), but mainly they are positive emotions. And to be honest having a good cry because the baby duck lost its mother, or something similar, can be oh so cathartic.

I WISH SOMEONE HAD TOLD ME ...
NOT TO GIVE UP "ME TIME"

Happy mummy = happy baby! I cannot stress this enough. If you are happy, refreshed (as can be with a newborn) and not stressed, your baby will benefit too. Your baby's well-being is directly linked to yours. So please try to retain some "me time". That means something different for everyone, but having some time where you can focus on yourself and do something you like is very important. It may just be going for a walk, seeing a movie with your partner or sitting by yourself enjoying a cup of tea. You probably don't want to spend time away from your gorgeous little munchkin but trust me, your baby will thank you for it. I know it is difficult to make the time, especially if you are breastfeeding two-hourly and don't have family around, but where there's a will, there's a way. And no, grocery shopping does not constitute "me time", don't even let your husband insinuate that ☺.

I WISH SOMEONE HAD TOLD ME ...
THERE IS A LOT OF SUPPORT

Among the chaos, you will find some kind faces. There will always be some mums who are going, or have gone, through the same things you have. They will totally get you and will have your back. The key is to keep an eye out and an ear open. While it can be tough in the beginning weeding out the honest from the honestly degrading, the cream rises to the top and you will most likely make life-long friends as you discuss very personal things with your new mum BFFs. It's wonderful! I don't know what I would do without my little support network of wonderful mums. You know who you are ☺. There is also a lot of great support from groups and organisations out there. You are not alone!

CONGRATULATIONS, YOU'RE A MUM!

I WISH SOMEONE HAD TOLD ME ...
THAT YOU ARE NOT A BAD MOTHER IF YOU DO NOT GET THAT IMMEDIATE RUSH OF LOVE FOR YOUR BABY

It is perfectly OK to not madly adore your baby the instant you lay eyes on him. I have heard from so many women that it took them a little while to fall in love with their child. Don't despair; it's totally normal and there is no time frame that it needs to happen in. A lot has happened: your body has gone through so much and hormones are ruling the roost. Be kind to yourself and allow yourself to connect with your baby in your own time. It is your journey with your little one, don't let anybody else dictate the steps.

I WISH SOMEONE HAD TOLD ME …
HOW INCREDIBLE SLEEP DEPRIVATION IS

I know you think you already know about the sleep deprivation, but trust me, you don't. Nothing can prepare you for the broken, and lack of, sleep. You may have been able to party until 6am in stilettos and then go straight into a full day of work, but you don't keep a rhythm like that for weeks or months (or years, if you're really unlucky) on end. Chances are your baby will though. The good news: your baby is adorable and you will forgive her night after night because she is just so darn cute. Oh, and you do kind of get used to the fragmented sleep. The bad news: there is a reason sleep deprivation is used as a form of torture; it messes with your mental and physical health. Please be kind to yourself and ask for help whenever possible. Still, you will be very tired all the time. No word of a lie, I have slept through the night maybe 10 times in the last six years. It is brutal! And nobody, and nothing, can prepare you for it.

I WISH SOMEONE HAD TOLD ME …
THAT PEOPLE BRAG ABOUT THE GOOD STUFF

Some people, who usually disguise themselves as "well-wishers" and "well-meaners", prefer to tell you the bad stuff and some can't help but gloat with the good. "My five-week old baby is feeding really well, sleeping through the night, always happy and makes his own lunch!" You will hear this stuff. Ignore it!!! And make new friends!

Because even if it is true… ha who am I kidding, it's not true. Ignore! Or even better… #unfriend. Take all stories, good and bad, with a grain of salt. You will hear lots of them but your journey into, and through, motherhood as unique as your baby is. Write your own story. And whatever you do, don't compare yourself. You're doing a great job!

I WISH SOMEONE HAD TOLD ME …
THAT MY MOTHERING WOULD BE JUDGED (OOPS, I MEAN I WISH SOMEONE HAD TOLD ME I WOULD RECEIVE A LOT OF "ADVICE")

Sadly, this is the reality of a new mum, more often than not. You can't seem to do anything without people, especially other mothers, throwing in their judgemental two cents. It can be extremely daunting when it is your first baby because, if you're like me, you may think that everyone else knows things better than you do. That could not be further from the truth – you are the best parent for your baby. Tell all the "do-gooders" (who really are do-badders) to get lost! I wish I had done that when I had my first because their constant judging, critiquing and "helping" made me feel completely inadequate. They may mean well, or they may not, but they will tell you what they think regardless of whether you ask them or not. Unfortunately, this often comes from other mothers which makes it even more frightening (don't let it get to you though). Thankfully (ha ha ha!) this is not limited to your first baby (I am still getting it now my third baby is two years old!).

So arm yourself with some good comebacks (polite and not so polite) and don't be afraid to use them.

I WISH SOMEONE HAD TOLD ME ...
THERE IS MORE THAN ONE WAY TO SKIN A CAT

There is more than one way to skin a cat! That was my mantra for the first few months, with my first-born, after I realised I was doing my head in worrying I was doing everything wrong. Early on I found that wherever I turned mothers seemed to be doing things differently. At the time I thought I was doing everything wrong but now I realise that it was just that... different. My son was healthy, happy, sleeping(ish), thriving and clean. I was most of those things too (yes, there were definitely days when showering didn't fit into the schedule) so there was nothing to worry about, yet I did. Lots! Because there is so much pressure and judgement (by you on yourself and sadly often by others) it is easy to fall into the trap of feeling like you are doing a bad job. If your baby is healthy and happy, that is all that matters. Trust me, once they are a bit older you'll realise it was worry for nothing. There is more than one way to skin a cat ☺.

I WISH SOMEONE HAD TOLD ME …
TO TRUST MY GUT

I can't stress this enough, please trust your instincts. You know best. It is your baby and your gut feeling is usually spot on. There is always a lot of information out there but when it comes to the crunch, trust yourself. You are doing great!

AND BABY MAKES THREE

I WISH SOMEONE HAD TOLD ME ...
I MAY DESPISE MY PARTNER

Why is my husband such a knob? Maybe he always was, maybe it's the hormones or maybe I was just completely sleep-deprived (or maybe it's just me!) but some things Hubs did in the beginning really annoyed me. Like not even wriggling when the baby woke (and then asking in the morning "did the baby sleep through the night?"). Or "suggesting" I eat a good meal for lunch because he had heard it's important when breastfeeding ("I will be lucky if I get to wee today, you numbnut, let alone make a sandwich!!"). Or generally just breathing too loudly. Yeah OK, it's probably a combination of hormones, sleep-deprivation, me being a knob and him being a knob (although he did often make me lunch and leave it in the fridge for me. Bless his cotton socks). Unfortunately, it is not restricted to your partner. If you have a mother/father/sibling/cousin/aunt that will be around a lot when you have a baby, they may cop some of it too. It sounds mean but I have always vowed to write the truth here, plus I have nothing left to hide and my dignity abandoned me long ago with my children's placentas. Truth be told, I know for a fact I am not the only one. You *will* be annoyed at one point or another. But this too shall pass, and rosier days will bless your little family. Plus, your partner may come in handy at some point down the track, so don't go smashing his face in just yet.

I WISH SOMEONE HAD TOLD ME...
EVEN THE STRONGEST RELATIONSHIP WILL PROBABLY TAKE A KNOCK WHEN YOU BRING YOUR BABY HOME

I think this is one of those topics that mothers *really* don't like talking about. Mainly because it admits a certain vulnerability i.e. your relationship is not bullet-proof. Hubs and I had a tough time when we brought Baby #1 home. I'll be the first to admit it, and I think if you ask him he will admit it too. Your whole life is turned upside down. What was just the two of you is now a crying, pooing, vomiting heap. But in my opinion it is sleep-deprivation and its friends that are the relationship killer, not the baby *per se*. A lack of sleep brings out the worst in everyone; it's no surprise it was used as a torture device. I am not a relationship expert but what helped us was communication. How cliché! I know it's the last thing you want to do after a day of new-found craziness, but it is imperative. Without words there is no unity, and without unity there is no family.

I WISH SOMEONE HAD TOLD ME...
I WOULD WORRY A LOT ABOUT MY BABY

Baby is not sleeping enough; baby is sleeping too much. Baby is not getting enough milk; baby is getting too much milk. Baby is not settling, baby doesn't like the bath, baby is posseting… the list goes on and on. Once your bundle is here, you will worry, stress, fuss and question everything. A lot. Most of us will do it, it is part of our make-up, I think. The good thing is that most of our worries are usually unfounded and our babies are actually doing great. Try not to fret, instead try to enjoy this special time.

I WISH SOMEONE HAD TOLD ME...
I MAY BE MORE FORGETFUL AFTER I HAVE MY BABY

You may know it as "baby brain" but it is also called "Mumnesia" ☺. So since there is a name for it, it must be real, right? Yes, it is very real! There have been studies done on the forgetfulness of new mums, and contrary to popular belief it is not just because you have so much on your mind. It is actually that those good old hormones, tiredness and stress are responsible for the memory loss by altering your brain size and chemistry. Thankfully this should only last the first few months of your baby's life (otherwise we would forever be needing several trips to the shops to remember what we went for). And on the upside there has been a study done that shows a mother's brain actually grows in certain areas that are linked to maternal behaviour (i.e. mothering!) when she has had her baby[15]. Just proves again how amazing and adaptable the human body (and brain) is.

I WISH SOMEONE HAD TOLD ME …
PEOPLE WILL ALWAYS ENQUIRE ABOUT THE NEXT BABY

A few women I have met told me they hadn't even left the hospital with their first baby when they were asked by "well-wishers" and "kind strangers" when the next baby would come. Some people are just crazy. Or dumb. Or both. Or they don't know what else to say but chances are "when is the next baby coming?" will get thrown at you a lot. I am not sure if it ever stops either (note to self: ask Hubs' cousin, who has six kids, if they still get asked). I have three beautiful, healthy kids, two boys and a girl (so the 'wouldn't you like a boy/girl' reason is out of the question) and people still ask me when #4 will come. My response: If I was 10 years younger blah blah blah… Other mums are not quite as courteous. I know one mum who says something along the lines of: "Have you ever seen Johnny's* wanger? If it wasn't so big maybe I would dare to have another baby but doing the deed with him is akin to childbirth itself." Love it!

* Johnny is an example name, of course.

I WISH SOMEONE HAD TOLD ME ...
THAT JUST BECAUSE YOU HAVE TROUBLE FALLING PREGNANT ONCE, DOESN'T MEAN YOU'LL HAVE TROUBLE THE NEXT TIME

I have spoken to quite a few women that had a lot of trouble falling pregnant, and when they finally gave birth to their much-wanted baby, they fell pregnant again almost immediately. Why? Because breastfeeding is *not* a contraceptive, ladies!!!! And because you are very fertile after you have a baby. But in all seriousness, I am thrilled that some women manage to get pregnant again so easily and I wanted to add this section to give all the couples, who had trouble falling pregnant in the past, hope. Just because it was difficult one time, doesn't mean it'll be hard the next.

I WISH SOMEONE HAD TOLD ME ...
THAT IT WOULD TAKE SO LONG TO FEEL NORMAL AGAIN

It can take a long time to feel "normal" again (in every sense of the word), no matter how you had your baby. It is hormone-driven and dependent on your delivery, support, subsequent children, mental state and all sorts of things. From a hormone point of view, it can take many, many months to get balanced again. The other aspects are dependent on your circumstance. It took me 18 months to feel "normal" again after having #3. There were many factors and I wish I had reminded myself that like everything it is a phase and it too shall pass. So please take it from me; you will feel "normal" again one day. For some women it is sooner, and some it takes a little while. Either way, it is OK. Just go with it, remind yourself everything will be fine and ask for help if you need it.

I WISH SOMEONE HAD TOLD ME…
IT WOULD TAKE SO LONG FOR MY HORMONES TO RE-STABILISE

Oh hormones, the bane of most women's existence. How can something serve such a great purpose and at the same time be so Grrrr! Your body is still going through lots of changes including breastfeeding, weaning and Aunt Flo making an avenging return… It can take a while for your hormones to get settled and re-stabilise completely. This can affect your general mood or your fertility i.e. conceiving another baby (which in itself can affect your general mood). I know many women who had trouble conceiving after their last baby because their menstrual cycle (*read*: hormones) were all over the place for a long time. I also know a mum who had a horrendous time around each menstrual period. It settled down for her when her baby was two years old. I am holding out hope for that time, as the period around my period is also quite torturous for me (and Hubs!), but it does seem to be getting better now Baby #3 is nearing her second birthday. I know that my friend and I are not alone in this category, so let's give three cheers and boos to hormones; our dream-maker and worst nightmare.

I WISH SOMEONE HAD TOLD ME ...
THAT SUBSEQUENT KIDS MAY NOT NECESSARILY BE EASIER

I mean easier in every possible regard. From pregnancy through to labour, the delivery, postpartum and the next 18 years. Each child is different, and just because you have done it before doesn't mean the next child won't throw you. Yes, you probably have more experience under your belt, but that doesn't count for much a lot of the time. I thought I had it pretty sussed when I became pregnant with my third baby. The pregnancy and birth were relatively straight-forward and I thought there wasn't much that could be thrown at me. I mean after all, I knew what I was doing, right? Wrooooong!!! Once my littlest one was in the world I realised I knew nothing, even though it had only been 21 months since my last baby and just over three years since my first. It took me a long time to get into a groove. People assumed I knew what I was doing, because I had two others, and all within three-and-a-half years, but they could not have been more wrong. Each child is different and each time you learn more. Remember I said that no mother has it all together. It is sooooooo true!!!

SEXY SEXY-TIME

I WISH SOMEONE HAD TOLD ME ...
THAT I MAY LIE TO MY PARTNER ABOUT WHEN WE CAN HAVE SEX AGAIN

OK, so there are exceptions to every rule but the majority of women will not feel like having sex once they have stopped bleeding (around six weeks postpartum). Whether you are physically, mentally or emotionally not ready, rest assured you are not alone. Many mums have told me that they may have told a little white lie to their partner saying their midwife actually advised 12 weeks of abstinence. One mum even said six months! Truth be told, if your partner ventured down "the other end" during or straight after your delivery, he probably will not want to have sex six weeks later anyway. But like I said there is an exception to every rule so keep the "I have a headache" excuse up your sleeve ☺.

I WISH SOMEONE HAD TOLD ME...
THAT IT CAN TAKE A WHILE FOR SEX TO FEEL GOOD AGAIN

Good on every level: physically, emotionally, spiritually... I could definitely have waited a looooong stretch to have sexy time with Hubs again. Especially after our first, who almost tore me in half, but after whom I also still carried a lot of extra weight. I also had the other wonderful (not!) "side effects" of just having had a baby that are mentioned in this book. So yeah, I was not one of those women who felt sexy. And sex, while being on the top of my To Do list, was not on top of my *Want* To Do list. The sheer thought of it scared the sh★t out of me (which would have been great if literal, because then at least I could have stopped worrying about doing a poo...). At first sex can be scary and it can feel strange or uncomfortable; a lot has changed in your body, physically and hormonally, so if it doesn't feel right at least you know you are not alone. It may never feel the same as pre-baby again but you just need to work with that. You never know, you may get a nice surprise and reaching orgasm in a position that was previously not doing it for you, now totally works. Too explicit? Oh come on, we all do it. I mean isn't that how our little bundles came into existence in the first place?

I WISH SOMEONE HAD TOLD ME...
I MAY LEAK BREASTMILK DURING SEX

I have spoken to women who when aroused, or orgasming, experience let-down. Of breastmilk that is, not let down of partner's performance ☺. Some people find this to be a huge turn on. And if you have a sterile container nearby you can collect some of the liquid gold while you're at it. Now that is multi-tasking! (I'm just kidding of course, don't collect milk, just have sex).

I WISH SOMEONE HAD TOLD ME...
I MAY LEAK URINE DURING SEX

On a not so arousing note (or maybe it is for you!?!), it is also possible to leak some pee while having sex. You may be fine on a day-to-day basis but the physical act of intercourse may cause a few drops to leak out. Strengthening your pelvic floor can help. Do your pelvic floor exercises, before baby, while pregnant and after baby. I cannot stress how important they are, so I wrote a whole paragraph about them. Have you read it? You will thank me when you're a grandma.

POST-BABY BODY
THINGS YOU MUST KNOW

I WISH SOMEONE HAD TOLD ME...
MY VAGINA WOULD NEVER LOOK THE SAME AGAIN

OK, let me warn you again: DO NOT look down there after you have given birth. There is a good reason for my warning; your vagina will never look the same again. Even if you had a really straight-forward birth, without tearing/grazing or anything else, let's not forget *a person came out of there*!!! And even after several weeks, oh let's be honest, even after years... your vagina will *never* look the same again. Enjoy it now look at it often and then say goodbye to it (yet another thing our children take from us ☺) when you hit the hospital in labour. By all means look at it at some point and check it out, but don't say I didn't warn you.

I WISH SOMEONE HAD TOLD ME ...
I MAY HAVE BACK ISSUES IF I HAVE AN EPIDURAL

There are no scientific links as such but if you ask around you will probably find quite a few mums that swear their epidural is the cause of their back problems. I have spoken to mums that say their backs were fine before they had an epidural and now, even months after having their baby, their backs crack at the site where the epidural was inserted. Some say they can't get a back massage because it feels like a lightning bolt is shooting through their body. Whereas some say they have constant back pain. It must be horrendous, and while this isn't the norm I thought it is worthy to mention, so you can be prepared for *everything*.

I WISH SOMEONE HAD TOLD ME ...
I WOULD FEEL PHANTOM PREGNANCY KICKS AFTER GIVING BIRTH

Phantom pregnancy kicks feel like your baby is still moving and "partying" inside your belly months after actually giving birth. I still felt these from time-to-time *16 months* after having my last baby. Upon investigating it further, there are women out there that feel them for years after giving birth. There is really no concrete explanation for this phenomenon but muscle and nerve memory may play a part. Or maybe your reproductive senses are playing with your emotions and trying to trick you into having another baby ☺. It is quite a nice feeling which can make you reminisce and somewhat miss the days when you did feel your baby move. But do you really want another baby? I'll stick with the phantom kicks, thank you very much.

I WISH SOMEONE HAD TOLD ME ...
THE SWELLING IN MY JOINTS COULD LAST FOR MONTHS

OK, so the puffy swelling that is due to the excess fluid and blood in your body should all be tinkled and sweated out several weeks after having your baby. Your face, ankles, feet and whatever else seems swollen should look "normal" in next to no time, and the discomfort should ease. If, however, you experience swelling in joints, such as the wrist, the resulting pain can last for many months. Carpal tunnel syndrome can develop during pregnancy and can, like it did for me after #1, get worse after you have your baby. I couldn't put any pressure on my wrists for many months. While this type of swelling can take time to resolve there are things you can do in the mean time to make it more bearable, such as a wrist splint.

OTHER IMPORTANT STUFF YOU MUST KNOW ABOUT YOUR POST-BABY BODY

I WISH SOMEONE HAD TOLD ME ...
THAT MY HAIR WILL NEVER BE THE SAME AGAIN

I hear a thousand tears drop to the tune of that one. I can vouch for this myself (I hear you sisters!!!). Say goodbye to those lustrous pregnancy locks. Once baby is here, you will firstly lose so much hair you'll be wondering if you'll have any left by the end of it. And then what is left will likely be nothing like the hair you had before. Blame those pesky hormones. Again! My gorgeous thick straight mane (*read*: slightly unmanageable and unruly but truly dead straight) turned into a pile of thick frizz. With each consecutive child my hair became wavier and wavier ("wavy" is what the hairdressers call it — it really is frizz). I always joke that if I had another eight kids I would probably have ringlets. No hairdresser ever finds that funny, but what they do seem to take great joy in is telling me that my hair will never go back to its pre-baby state and I will be a frizz, ah I mean wave, ball forever.

I WISH SOMEONE HAD TOLD ME ...
ABOUT THE SKIN CHANGES

Those bloody hormones again!!! If you have never had acne, dry skin or spider veins in your life, post-pregnancy may be the time you first meet them. On the flip-side if you had bad skin while pregnant this could all suddenly clear up once bub is born. It's crazy! The good news is that if you have bad skin post-baby, it should resolve once your hormones are balanced again (cue: happy face). As for the mask of pregnancy, the dark discoloration of the skin around the eyes, cheeks, forehead and sometimes mouth? It generally fades sometime after you give birth, although apparently it will never go away completely (cue: sad face).

I WISH SOMEONE HAD TOLD ME ...
THAT MY MIDSECTION WILL NEVER BE THE SAME AGAIN

Take a photo of your tummy now. Well, ideally before you fall pregnant but for most reading this that is probably too late. So do it now. Because even if you are lucky enough to have a flat stomach again one day your belly button will never look the same. Mine is a bit like a dehydrated doughnut. It resembles a once-round shape but it's kind of saggy and the skin around it may in actual fact belong to my 99-year-old grandmother in-law. That can be said for my whole midsection actually. Having gained 20+kg with each child and then losing it, my tummy resembles that of a Shar Pei (think Rolly the wrinkly dog). It does tone back a little over time but for me if I am upside down it is wrinkle city.

I WISH SOMEONE HAD TOLD ME...
THAT MY WHOLE BODY WILL NEVER BE THE SAME AGAIN

Your midsection is not the only thing that will change shape (and stay that way!), you will hear that many women, if not all, find that their whole body shape changes in one way or another. That is not necessarily a bad thing. I prefer my body now to the one I had pre-babies. And many other women do too. It may mean that you need a whole new wardrobe of clothes though (diddums!) because your new shape is just not suited to your old clothes. This may also go for your feet. A lot of women's feet remain the size they grow to during pregnancy. So add shoe shopping to your list of things to do. Yay, sounds great! Except of course for your boobs... Boooooo! I don't think there are many women that prefer the snooker-ball-in-a-sock look to perky or at least non-sucked-dry breasts. Luckily there are some very awesome bras on the market these days. Note: also add bra shopping to the list of things to do.

I WISH SOMEONE HAD TOLD ME ...
TO HOLD OFF BUYING BRAS

OK, so here is a tip, don't buy too many maternity bras when you are pregnant. Yes, they are super comfy but your boobs will grow *a lot* as your pregnancy progresses. And when your milk comes in... well, your fun bags will explode! Same goes for bras post-pregnancy and/or breastfeeding. Don't buy anything nice for months after you stop breastfeeding. You will still produce milk for a while even if your baby has fully weaned (it's really kinda weird, actually) so your boobs will still continue to shrink over time i.e. deflate! I learnt this the hard way after #1 weaned. Stopped breastfeeding, bought four *gorgeous* bras. Wore them only a hand-full of times because before I knew it my rack-of-plenty was less than a hand-full (cue: very sad face and empty wallet).

FINAL THOUGHTS

I know this may seem like a long list of negatives with just a few positives thrown in for good measure. That isn't deliberate. My intention of researching and writing this book was to tell you the things nobody tells you about. Fortunately, positive things are discussed frequently, so you don't need to hear them again. While it may seem like labour, delivery, matrescence and the first few weeks of motherhood are a horrible experience, the truth is they are amazing and truly magical. When you give birth to your baby you are transformed; you are a mum! Holding your baby in your arms is the most wonderful feeling in the world. Like labour, you can't describe it. You have to experience it. I spent close to six years researching and writing this book, and as you can see, I came across some pretty gnarly stories. But none of them put me off having three kids.

I hope that this book will make your experience a little less daunting, because you now know *all* that I, and one thousand other mums, know. Or at the very least I hope you feel like you are not alone. Because you are not. Welcome to The Secret Mothers Club!

A GIFT FROM ME TO YOU!

Thank you so much for taking the time to read my book.

I hope you feel empowered with knowledge and ready for your transition into motherhood.

If you enjoyed the book, I would very much appreciate a review on Goodreads, www.DrJen.com.au/reviews, Amazon, Facebook, or all four ☺

MY FREE GIFT TO YOU!

Take the next step in preparing yourself for motherhood

DOWNLOAD MY MATRESCENCE PREPARATION MINI COURSE

It's totally FREE and available at:
www.DrJen.com.au/freebie

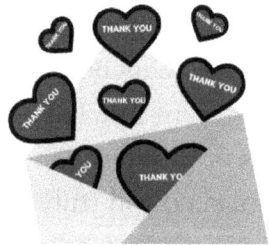

As a thank you, and to get you off to a great start in your motherhood transformation, matrescence, I would like to give you my FREE matrescence preparation mini course.

Download it today at www.DrJen.com.au/freebie

REFERENCES

[1] Gaskin IM (2003) Going backwards: the concept of 'pasmo'. Pract Midwife 6(8):34-7.

[2] Postel T (2013) Childbirth climax: The revealing of obstetrical orgasm. Sexologies 22(4):165-8.

[3] What to Expect. Childbirth stage 2: pushing the baby out <http://www.whattoexpect.com/pregnancy/labor-and-delivery/childbirth-stages/pushing-and-delivery.aspx> Accessed 29 February 2016.

[4] American Pregnancy Association. Crowning <http://americanpregnancy.org/labor-and-birth/crowning/> Accessed 29 February 2016.

[5] Craciunas L, Sajid MS, Ahmed AS (2014) Chewing gum in preventing postoperative ileaus in women undergoing caesarean section: a systematic review and meta-analysis of randomised controlled trials. BJOG 121(7):793-9.

[6] Ledari ML, Barat S, Delavar MA, Banihosini SZ, Khafri S (2013) Sugar-free gum reduces ileaus after caesarean section in nulliparous women: a randomized clinical trial. Iran Red Crescent Med J 15(4):330-334.

[7] Merriam-Webster Medical Dictionary. Referred Pain <http://www.medicinenet.com/script/main/art.asp?articlekey=34151> Accessed 14 March 2016.

[8] Blackburn, ST (2013) Maternal, fetal and neonatal physiology: a clinical perspective, 4th edition. USA: Elsevier Saunders. Pp 658-9.

[9] Hedayati H, Parsons J, Crowther CA (2003) Rectal analgesia for pain from perineal trauma following childbirth (Review). Cochrane pregnancy and childbirth group. Cochrane library 2003, issue 3.

[10] Swain JE, Tasgin E, Mayes LC, Feldman R, Constable RT, Leckman JF (2008) Maternal brain response to own baby-cry is affected by caesarean section delivery. J Child Psychol Psychiatry 49(10):1042-52.

[11] Pelvic Pain and Rehab. C-Section scar: problems and solutions <http://www.pelvicpainrehab.com/pelvic-pain/2000/c-section-scar-problems-and-solutions/> Accessed 15 March 2016.

[12] Black Dog Institute. Postnatal depression <http://www.blackdoginstitute.org.au/public/depression/inpregnancypostnatal/postnataldepressionpnd.cfm> Accessed 7 March 2016.

[13] Australian Breastfeeding Association. The let-down reflex <https://www.breastfeeding.asn.au/bf-info/early-days/let-down-reflex> Accessed 14 March 2016.

[14] Perinatal anxiety and depression Australia. Postnatal anxiety and depression <http://www.panda.org.au/practical-information/about-postnatal-depression/28-postnatal-depression?showall=&start=1> Accessed 7 March 2016.

[15] The Telegraph. "Baby brain' really does exist, say scientists <http://www.telegraph.co.uk/news/science/science-news/10812090/Baby-brain-really-does-exist-say-scientists.html> Accessed 15 March 2016.

DR JENNIFER HACKER PEARSON PhD

Dr Jen has three kids, one husband, two dogs, one cat and a bird.

She holds a PhD in Medicine (Neuroscience and Pharmacology), a degree in Psychotherapy, and is an accredited meditation teacher.

I Wish Someone Had Told Me... is her debut book, although she has been published in many peer-reviewed scientific journals, such as *Nature Neuroscience*.

Dr Jen is passionate about creating educational and practical neuroscientific and neurocognitive-based support for mothers during matrescence (becoming a mother) by running online courses, writing, hosting her podcast *Mama Unleashed!* and speaking to women in workshops and on stages, worldwide.

Dr Jen's business focuses on educating women about how becoming a mother, aka entering matrescence, changes women, in particular their brain and mind, and how you can use this very transformational time to teach your brain and mind to thrive in motherhood.

You can find out more about Dr Jen and her work at
www.DrJen.com.au

Or on Facebook, Instagram and YouTube
@DrJenHackerPearson

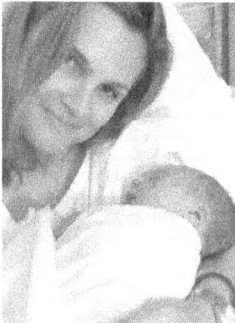

This is the photo I posted on social media that set the wheels in motion for this book.

www.ingramcontent.com/pod-product-compliance
Lightning Source LLC
Chambersburg PA
CBHW060309220326
41598CB00027B/4276